DENTISTRY AND ORAL SCIENCES

A COMPENDIUM OF PRINCIPLES AND PRACTICES OF LASER BIOPHOTONICS IN ORAL MEDICINE

DENTISTRY AND ORAL SCIENCES

Additional books and e-books in this series can be found
on Nova's website under the Series tab.

DENTISTRY AND ORAL SCIENCES

A COMPENDIUM OF PRINCIPLES AND PRACTICES OF LASER BIOPHOTONICS IN ORAL MEDICINE

FAKIR MOHAN DEBTA
EKAGRATA MISHRA
AND
NEHA PATYAL

nova
science publishers
New York

DOI: https://doi.org/10.52305/EWUD9733

NOTICE TO THE READER

Library of Congress Cataloging-in-Publication Data

ISBN: 978-1-68507-441-8

Published by Nova Science Publishers, Inc. † New York

Dedicated to all the times, places and people which/who are a source of perpetual inspiration...

Dedicated to You, The Reader...

Contents

LIST OF FIGURES

LIST OF TABLES

FOREWORD

The textbook titled "A Compendium of Principles and Practices of Laser Biophotonics in Oral Medicine" provides an essential resource for the learning of laser dentistry. It adds to the repertoire of books on the subject and lends our students a useful adjuvant to face any examination, both objectively and subjectively.

Dr. Fakir Mohan Debta has thoughtfully and meticulously produced this admirable compilation which is an aid to the judicious student in pursuit of a ready reckoner or easy reference to the practice of lasers in dentistry. His co-authors, Dr. Ekagrata Mishra and Dr. Neha Patyal, have provided their valuable inputs and additions to develop this work as a valuable and erudite discourse on the subject.

Laser dentistry serves to present a more accurate, precise and painless approach to the practice of dentistry and lends the profession an adjuvant facet of specialization directed towards better care of our patients.

Prof. Dr. Fakir Mohan Debta and his team of authors strive to exemplify the scientific and clinical aspects of laser dentistry through their laborious efforts and I'm sure it will benefit the multitude of students and teachers who hope to further fathom the depths of learning.

Sincerely,

Alex Mathews Muruppel
Principal, Rajas Dental College & Hospital,
Kanyakumari, Tamilnadu, India
Professor (A.C) International Faculty Panel, Department of Integrated Surgical and Diagnostic Sciences, & Academic Director for India, Universita degli Studi di Genova, Italy
Fellow of Pierre Fauchard Academy
Nobel Biocare Fellow in Implantology

PREFACE

This book entitled *A Compendium of Principles and Practices of Laser Biophotonics in Oral Medicine.* has been compiled with an overall appraisal with regard to laser, its construction, operation and implementation as an innovative diagnostic, therapeutic and adjunctive tool in the field of oral medicine and oral diagnostics, and allied applications.

The contents herein have been segregated into 14 chapters, giving an overview of the perspectives discussed, ensuring ease of navigation and providing a simple and logical nexus of guideposts. A brief content analysis is presented hereafter.

Chapter 1 - "Introduction," is an introduction to biophotonics technology with Laser (Light Amplification by the Stimulated Emission of Radiation) being one of the most important inventions of the twentieth century in biophotonic technology and how due to their remarkable properties, lasers are finding applications in all aspects of human endeavors. This chapter briefly acquaints us with the advent of laser dentistry, its advantages and disadvantages, and its role in various fields of dentistry with special focus on its use in the field of oral medicine and oral diagnostics. This chapter serves as a prelude to the discussions that follow.

Chapter 2 - "History of Lasers," discusses the milestone achievements and their pioneers in the field of lasers and laser dentistry in chronologic order.

Chapter 3 - "The Laser Device," discusses the basic construction and working of lasers. This chapter also gives an overview about the generic classification of lasers based on the active medium incorporated into its design, currently available visible spectrum dental lasers, currently available invisible spectrum dental lasers and various laser delivery systems.

Chapter 4 - "The Laser Beam," presents the various properties of a laser beam with regard to its chromaticity, coherence, directionality, focusability and other properties of practical relevance.

Chapter 5 - "Laser-Tissue Interactions," elucidates how the potential for laser–tissue interaction forms the basis of the usefulness of predictable employment of laser photonic energy. All potential, possible laser-tissue interactions, their variation with power density and temperature have been discussed.

Chapter 6 - "Laser Terminologies and Dosimetry," presents various laser parameters that define a laser unit and/or its properties in a tabular and graphical format.

Chapter 7 - "Laser Hazards and Contraindications," provides a risk stratification of lasers along with potential risks and hazards associated with laser use. A logical appraisal of contraindications of lasers has been done under 3 groups-justified, doubtful and erroneous.

Chapter 8 - "Laser Safety," safety is an integral part of any device or instrument before, during and after use. Various factors for laser safety and safety protocols laid down by apex regulatory authorities have been discussed.

Chapters 9, 10, 11, 12 and 13, gives a comprehensive account of practical applications of laser in contemporary oral medicine and diagnostics.

Chapter 9 - "Low power lasers and their applications," has been subdivided as follows for ease and clarity of discussion: "Introduction to Low Power Lasers" (9.1), "Cellular mechanisms of Photobiomodulation"

(9.2), "Principles of Photodynamic Therapy" (9.3), "Lasers in Recurrent Apthous Ulcerations" (9.4), "Lasers in Burning Mouth Syndrome" (9.5), "Lasers in Temporomandibular Joint Disorders" (9.6), "Lasers in Lymphatic Drainage of Oedema" (9.7), "Lasers in Herpes Infections" (9.8) and "Other applications of Low Level Laser Therapy" (9.9). Sub-sections 9.2 and 9.3 provide a theoretical premise of applications of low level lasers. Subsequent sub-sections (9.4-9.8) discuss most common practical implications of low level lasers. Section 9.9 summarizes other potential applications of low level lasers namely, Alveolar osteitis, neurosensory recovery after injury to inferior alveolar nerve, Bell's palsy, Trigeminal neuralgia, Post-herpetic neuralgia, oral lesions in Pemphigus, oral lesions in Steven-Johnsons syndrome and Toxic epidermal necrolysis, oral mucositis, Bisphosphonate induced Osteoradionecrosis and Pericoronitis. Applications of low level lasers in oral potentially malignant disorders like oral lichen planus have been discussed separately in Chapter 10 dedicated specifically to OPMD's.

Chapter 10 - "Lasers in Oral Potentially Malignant Disorders". Oral cancers may be preceded by oral potentially malignant disorders which are recognizable mucosal diseases harboring increased risk of development of squamous cell carcinoma; these lesions hence provide a therapeutic window for vigilant clinicians to intervene. Lasers can be used as dependable equipment to therapeutically address these lesions. This chapter has been divided into the following five sections: "Introduction to Lasers in Oral Potentially Malignant Disorders" (10.1), "Lasers in Oral Leukoplakia" (10.2), "Lasers in Actinic Chelitis" (10.3), "Lasers in Oral Erythroplakia" (10.4) and "Lasers in Oral Lichen Planus" (10.5).

Chapter 11 - "Surgical lasers and their applications" sheds light on the role of lasers as an optical-knife with their pros and cons measured against conventional scalpel surgery. This chapter has been discussed under the following subsections: "Introduction to Surgical Lasers" (11.1), "Lasers in Oral Fibromas" (11.2), "Lasers in Oral Squamous Papillomas" (11.3), "Lasers in Oral Lipomas" (11.4), "Lasers in Oral Pyogenic

Granulomas" (11.5), "Lasers in Oral Vascular Lesions" (11.6) and "Lasers in Salivary Gland Pathosis" (11.7).

Chapter 12 - "Laser Diagnostics." Lasers hold a commendable position in current and future role in diagnostics as a novel tool. This is elucidated by discussing: "Lasers in Caries Detection" (12.1), "Laser Doppler Flowmetry" (12.2), "Laser Optothermal Radiometry" (12.3), "Optical Coherence Tomography" (12.4), and "Confocal Laser Endomicroscopy" (12.5), "Photodynamic Diagnosis" (12.6), "Laser Spectroscopy" (12.7) and "Laser Flowcytometry" (12.8).

Chapter 13 - "Miscellaneous Applications of Lasers." This chapter provides a brief run through the following potential applications of lasers: "Lasers in Dentinal Hypersensitivity" (13.1), "Lasers in Sinusitis" (13.2), "Lasers in Somatosensory Tinnitus" (13.3), "Laser Acupuncture" (13.4), "Antimicrobial Photodynamic Therapy" (13.5), "Lasers in Caries Prevention" (13.6), "Laser Induced Tooth Analgesia" (13.7), "Lasers in Sterilization" (13.8) and "Lasers in other fields of Dentistry" (13.9).

Lastly, "Conclusion." "To know is to use. To understand is to empower…" This section provides a few remarks of closure to the compendium, enumerating its promising future applications in the field of oral medicine and diagnostics.

ACKNOWLEDGMENTS

"It is in collaboration that the nature of art is truly revealed."

We extend our sincere humilities and gratitude to the following people, whose constructive criticism and relentless support have helped mould this project from its very infancy. Dr. Jayanta Kumar Dash, Dr. Kunal Agarwal, Dr. Shreeyam Mohapatra, Dr. Shweta Mishra, Dr. Rupsa Nayana Rout, Dr. Pinali Das, Dr. Priyanka Debta, Dr. Pooja Bohidar, Dr. B Krishnapriya, and Dr. Prashant Goyal.

We would like to acknowledge the publisher, editors, and support staff at Nova Science Publishers, who have been an indispensable support during various stages of developing and producing the volume.

We are extremely humbled to receive a generous and thoughtful contribution to the foreword section of this book by Dr. Alex Mathews Muruppel.

List of Abbreviations

AC	Alternating Current
ALA	5-aminolevulinic acid
AlGaAs	Aluminum Gallium Arsenide
ANIT	Atraumatic and Non Invasive Treatment
ANSI	American National Standards Institute
AP-1	Activator Protein-1
APC	Antigen Presenting Cells
aPDT	Antimicrobial Photodynamic Therapy
ATF/CREB	Activating Transcription Factor/cAMP-response element-binding protein
BMS	Burning Mouth Syndrome
CCD	Charged Coupled Device
CDRH	Center for Devices and Radiological Health
CFU	Colony Forming Units
CLE	Confocal Laser Endomicroscopy
Cox	Cytochrome c oxidase
CR	Complete Remission
CTP	Connective Tissue Papilla
CW	Continuous Wave
DC	Direct Current
DIFOTI	Digital Imaging Fibre-Optic Transillumination

EPT	Electric Pulp Test
ES-SCC	Early-stage Squamous Cell Carcinoma
FDA	Food and Drug Administration
FD-LUM	Fournier Domain Luminescence
FD-OTR	Optothermal Radiometry
FOTI	Fibre-Optic Trans Illumination
GaAs	Gallium Arsenide
GP	Gated Pulse
HDL	High Density Lipoprotein
HIF-1	Hypoxia-inducible factor
HLLT	High-Level Laser Therapy
HMG	High-Mobility Group proteins
HPV	Human papilloma virus
HSV	Herpes Simplex virus
InGaAs	Indium Gallium Arsenide
InGaAsP	Indium Gallium Arsenide Phosphate
IR	Infrared
KTP	Potassium Titanyl Phosphate
LASER	Light Amplification by Stimulated Emission of Radiation
LDF	Laser Doppler Flowmetry
LDL	Low Density Lipoprotein
LED	Light Emitting Diode
LIBS	Laser-induced breakdown spectroscopy
LLLT	Low Level Laser Therapy
LPIRC	Low Power Infra Red laser
LPL	Low Power Laser
MAL	Methyl 5-aminolevulinate
MASCC	Multinational Association of Supportive Care in Cancer
MASER	Microwave Amplification by Stimulated Emission of Radiation
MCM	Mini-Chromosome Maintenance proteins
MEMS	Microelectromechanical System

m-MPQ	Modified McGill pain questionnaire
MPE	Maximum Permissible Exposure
Nd:YAG	Neodymium Doped Yttrium Aluminum Garnet
NFB	Nuclear Factor B
NO	Nitric Oxide
NTCLT	Non-ablative Non-thermal Cardon-dioxide Laser Therapy
OCT	Optical Coherence Tomography
OD	Optical Density
OHIP-CRO 14	Oral Health Impact Profile Questionnaires (14 items) in Croatian language
OHSA	Occupational Safety and Health Administration
OL	Oral Leukoplakia
OLP	Oral Lichen Planus
OPMDs	Oral Potentially Malignant Disorders
OSP	Oral squamous papilloma
OTR	Optothermal Radiometry
pO_2	tissue partial oxygen pressure
PACT	Photodynamic Antimicrobial Chemotherapy
PAD	Photoactivated Disinfection
PBM	Photobiomodulation
PDD	Photodynamic Diagnosis
PDI	Photodynamic Inactivation
PDT	Photodynamic Therapy
PG-E2	Prostaglandin E2
PHN	Post Herpetic Neuralgia
PLGA	poly (lactic-co-glycolic)
p-n	Positive-Negative junction
PPIX	Protoporphyrin IX
PS-OCT	Polarization-sensitive optical coherence tomography
PVL	Proliferative Verrucous Leukoplakia
QLF	Quantitative Light-induced Fluorescence
RAU	Recurrent Aphthous Ulcer

Ref-1	Redox Factor-1
RF	Radiofrequency
ROS	Reactive Oxygen Species
SCC	Squamous Cell Carcinoma
SD-OCT	Spectral Domain-Optical Coherence Tomography
SS-OCT	Swept Source- Optical Coherence Tomography
TD-OCT	Time domain-Optical Coherence Tomography
TEA	Transversely Excited Atmosphere
TMD	Temporomandibular Dysfunction
UV	Ultraviolet
VAS	Visual Analog Scale
WD-SCC	Well-differentiated Squamous Cell Carcinoma
WHO	World Health Organization
YAG	Yttrium Aluminum Garnet
YAP	Yttrium Aluminum Perovskite
YSGG	Yttrium Scandium Gallium Garnet

Chapter 1

INTRODUCTION

"And God said: Let there be light, and there was light. God saw that the light was good..."

(Holy Bible, Genesis 1:3) [1]

The word light has been used for many centuries, including biblical references, such as in the beginning sentences of the Book of Genesis [1]. The knowledge that light is beneficial and may lead to a cure does not belong exclusively to our time; Greek and ancient Egyptian doctors practised cures by exposure to sunlight. However, it was in the past century that one of the great technological advancements emerged as a revolution [2].

Photonics is a light-based optical technology that is considered the leading technology for the new millennium. The science of light generation, manipulation, transmission, and measurement is known as *photonics*. The application of photonics technologies and principles to medicine and life sciences is known as *biophotonics* [3]. During the last 50 years, there have been many breakthroughs in photonics that laid the foundation for its wide range of applications in health care. Most applications of photonics in health care were based on various types of light and different types of photon-tissue interactions. The application of photonics-based techniques offers several specific advantages such as rapidity, sensitivity, specificity, inexpensive and non-invasive [3, 4]. It has been observed that many diseases of the mouth are accompanied by characteristic changes in the tissue structure. Some typical examples include dental caries, non-carious lesions in teeth, gingivitis, periodontitis, precancerous lesions, and tumours of the oral tissues. Dentistry has traditionally depended on contemporary science and technology for improvement in diagnostic tools and advancement in treatment options. The current dental practice has been emphasizing more on early diagnosis and prevention of common oral diseases and conserving tooth structure as much as possible during restorative procedures. Thus, Atraumatic and Non-Invasive Treatment (ANIT) modalities have been the key thrust in dentistry today [5]. Keeping in mind the tremendous potential of optical technology to provide highly sensitive tissue information non-invasively, and the ability to induce localized and specific tissue changes, this should be the foremost technology to embrace for advancement in dentistry [6].

Laser (Light Amplification by the Stimulated Emission of Radiation) is one of the most important inventions of twentieth-century biophotonic technology [3]. Due to its remarkable properties it is finding applications in all aspects of human endeavour - industry, medicine, defence, basic research, and even home entertainment. The diverse use of lasers can be put in perspective by noting that while lasers are being used to generate the highest temperatures on earth, as high as millions of degrees Kelvin, as available in the core of the sun, they are also being used to generate the lowest temperatures on earth, as low as a few nano Kelvin [4]. Similarly, while lasers are being used to weld sheets of metal, they are also being used to weld the delicate layers of the retina. With such a versatile tool in hand, remarkable developments have occurred in the field of dental medicine and dental practice.

The introduction of lasers in dentistry, in the 1960s, by Miaman, led to continuous research in the various applications of lasers in dental practice [7]. There are two scenarios: on one hand, there are hard lasers, such as, Carbon dioxide (CO_2), Neodymium Yttrium Aluminium Garnet

(Nd: YAG), and Er:YAG, which offer both hard tissue and soft tissue applications, but have limitations due to high costs and potential for thermal injury to the tooth pulp, whereas, on the other hand in cold or soft lasers, based on the semiconductor diode devices, which are compact, low-cost devices used predominantly for applications, are broadly termed as low-level laser therapy (LLLT) or 'biostimulation.' [8, 9]. On account of the ease, efficiency, specificity, comfort, and cost over the conventional modalities, lasers are indicated for a wide variety of procedures in dental practice.

Laser light in dentistry is a unique, non-ionizing form of electromagnetic radiation that can be employed as a controlled source of tissue stimulation, cutting, or ablation, depending on specific parameters of wavelength, power, and the target tissue. Lasers have a myriad of hard and soft tissue applications in various specialized fields of dentistry. Uses in preventive, aesthetic, and restorative dentistry include selective caries removal, cavity preparation, treatment of non-carious cervical lesions, dental bleaching, hypersensitivity, etc. Most common endodontic applications include root canal sterilization using antimicrobial photodynamic therapy and high power laser-assisted apical surgeries. Lasers can also be used for surgical and non-surgical treatments of periodontal diseases and aesthetic treatment procedures of the periodontium. This modern age scalpel or optical knife can be used in various soft tissue Oral surgeries. It finds its application in fields of bone biomodulation, Implantology, and Orthodontics [8, 9].

In the field of Oral Medicine, Lasers have a multitude of preventive, therapeutic, and adjunctive applications in delivering a stage of tissue management conducive to achieving a completed hard or soft tissue procedure. Applications in clinical scenarios like Orofacial pain, Temporomandibular joint disorders, potentially malignant disorders of the oral mucosa, Herpes, recurrent aphthous ulcers, Burning mouth syndrome, nerve repair, laser and antimicrobial photodynamic therapies in cancer patients, non-neoplastic proliferative lesions of oral soft tissue, vascular lesions, have shown promising results. Lasers also aid in the optical enhanced diagnosis of oral lesions using fluorescence, coherence, and spectroscopic techniques [10-12].

Laser dental care can be advantageous in being quicker and more efficient along with markedly reduced pain, lack of bleeding, the minimal need of anaesthesia, minimal postoperative discomfort, patients can resume their daily activities shortly after the treatment is rendered, with improved compliance in the geriatric and paediatric population. But no technology is absolute and fail-safe [11]. Limitations of lasers include relatively high cost, requirement of training, modifications of clinical technique. The patient must be given appropriate postoperative instructions to correctly care for the area during healing. No single wavelength will optimally treat all dental diseases. The clinician must prevent the overheating the tissue while attempting to complete a procedure, carbonization, and production of the laser plume. Most technicalities can be corrected with experience and adherence to laser safety protocols [10].

This compendium aims to discuss the concepts of laser physics and its biological consequence on oral tissues, the advent of laser revolution into the dental practice, and applications of laser biophotonics in dentistry with special orientation to its preventive, therapeutic, and adjunctive use in oral medicine. The first step towards efficient laser dentistry is to seek objective information on all aspects of the instrument and its uses. If all aspects are weighed out, recommendations and protocols followed judiciously, lasers can be high quality, minimally invasive, comfortable, and patient-friendly equipment with favourable and expedited results.

Chapter 2

HISTORY OF LASERS

- Ibn al-Haytham, Persian mathematician, scientist, and philosopher, in his *Book of Optics* (1021), described light as being composed of a stream of tiny particles that travels in straight lines and bounce off objects that they strike [13].
- Pierre Gassendi, a French philosopher, scientist, astronomer, and mathematician, described his particle theory of light (published in 1658 as part of the six volumes of the *Opera Omnia*) [14].
- Newton proposed the theory of particle dynamics, which later was used to describe the behaviour of particles reacting to the influence of arbitrary forces [15].
- In 1665, English scientist Robert Hooke suggested his wave theory of light, likening the spread of light vibrations to that of waves in water: 'every pulse or vibration of the luminous body will generate a sphere, which will continually increase, and grow bigger, just after the same manner (though infinitely swifter) as the waves or rings on the surface of the water do swell into bigger and bigger circles about a point.' [16]
- On Dec. 14, 1900, German physicist Max Planck delivered a lecture before the German Physical Society, in which he theorized that light consisted of discrete and indivisible packets

of radiant energy that he named *quanta*. He described the elemental unit of energy (E), as E = hv, where *h* is a constant of nature with the dimension of action (= energy × time, 6.626 × 10–34 joule second), subsequently called Planck's constant, and *v* is the frequency of radiation. Planck's theory was published late in 1900. [17]

- Eleven years later, British physicist Ernest Rutherford contributed to quantum theory when he postulated a planetary model of the atom [18].
- When the quantum theory was in its nascent stage, Albert Einstein made significant contributions. First, in 1905, Einstein developed his light quantum theory: 'In the propagation of a light ray emitted from a point source, the energy is not distributed continuously over ever-increasing volumes of space, but consists of a finite number of energy quanta localized at points of space that move without dividing, and can be absorbed or generated as complete units' [19].
- American physicist Charles H. Townes, at Columbia University, did pioneering work in laser development. In 1951, in Washington, DC, Townes proposed the concept of a *maser,* an acronym he and his students coined for *m*icrowave *a*mplification by *s*timulated *e*mission of *r*adiation. He indicated that the 'primary object of the work that led to the maser was to get shorter wavelengths so that we could do better spectroscopy in a new spectral region.' [20].
- While on sabbatical from Columbia University in 1955, Townes worked with French physicist Alfred Kastler in Paris. Kastler developed the technique of "optical pumping," a process in which light is used to raise (or pump) electrons from a lower to a higher energy level, as a new way to excite materials for microwave spectroscopy. Townes recognized that optical pumping might excite the optical energy levels necessary for an optical maser [21]

- American physicist, Gordon Gould, a Columbia graduate student in 1957, asked whether optical pumping could excite light emission. He recorded his ideas in nine handwritten pages of a laboratory notebook, with the first page titled "Some rough calculations on the feasibility of a LASER: Light Amplification by Stimulated Emission of Radiation," the first time the term *laser* was used [22].
- On July 7, 1960, Maiman identified five potential uses for the laser: 1. The first true amplification of light. 2. A tool to probe matter for basic research. 3. High-power beams for space communications. 4. Increasing the number of available communication channels. 5. Concentrating light for industry, chemistry, and medicine [7].
- Pioneering examinations to find new and effective methods of removing caries, by interactions of ruby laser energy with tooth structure, were reported in the mid-1960s. Investigators discovered that the ruby laser could vaporize caries, but that the high-energy densities caused irreversible necrotic changes in the pulpal tissues [23].
- Years later, the development of erbium (Er) laser wavelengths, better suited to the clinical requirements for cavity preparation without the detrimental effects on pulp, led to further investigations [23].
- Early intraoral soft tissue investigations were conducted using the ruby laser. The development of the CO_2 laser and its ability to ablate soft tissue with minimal haemorrhage led to studies in oral surgery. Other groups followed up with soft tissue studies involving the Nd:YAG laser [8, 9].
- Dental practitioner, Dr. Goldman, became the first to design a laser specifically for general dentistry [24].
- Currently, several laser wavelengths are used in oral surgery and dentistry, including CO_2, Nd:YAG, argon, various diode wavelengths, two erbium wavelengths, and potassium titanyl phosphate (KTP) [8, 9].

Chapter 3

THE LASER DEVICE

All laser devices are fundamentally composed of an energy source and an optical resonator (Figure 1) [25].

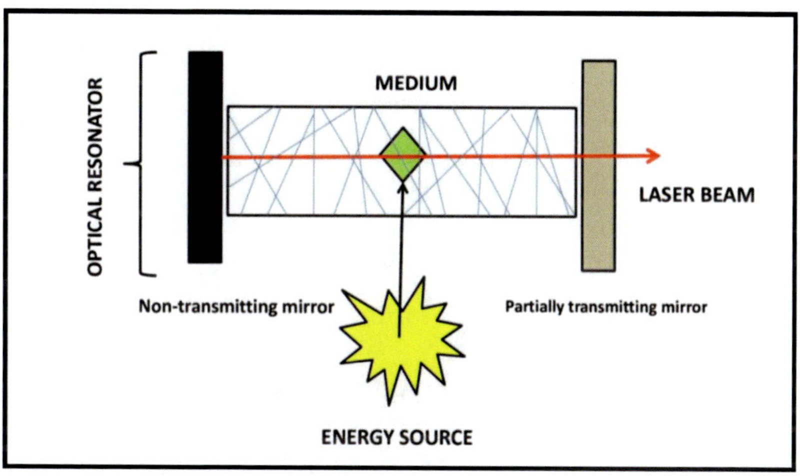

Figure 1. Laser components. The energy source will stimulate the electrons of a certain medium that will release photons that will be reflected on a non-transmitting mirror and be released as a collimated beam through the partially transmitting mirror.

a. The *energy source* is used to initially move the electrons into an excited state to ultimately generate the photons. This energy source can constitute of lamps, electrical current, or even other lasers [25]
b. The *optical resonator* is composed of the *medium* that is enclosed within *a tube that has 2 mirrors*: one mirror is completely opaque, and the other mirror is partially opaque, hence, partially transmissible. The medium can be in the form of a solid, liquid crystal (a liquid crystal has an atomic organization that is intermediate between a solid and a liquid), liquid, or gas. It is the medium that determines the wavelength and identification of the laser [10].

For dentistry, there are two basic types of lasers [8, 9]:

a. One that operates as a semiconductor and is compact - Diode Laser
b. One that has distinct components that, when assembled, occupy a larger footprint- encompasses all other lasers

Both of these types share common features—an *active medium*, a *pumping mechanism*, and a *resonator*. In addition, a cooling system, controls, and a delivery system complete the laser device.

3.1. Active Medium

Lasers are generically named as per the active medium (Table 1, 2). It is the material that is being stimulated, contained, or housed at the centre or core of the laser, termed the optical cavity. Upon absorption of photonic energy, the atoms (or molecules) of the active medium begin to spontaneously emit and under the right conditions, the process of stimulated emission will begin. Common materials for dental lasers can be broadly grouped into one of three types: a container of *gas*, a *solid-state crystal*, or a *semiconductor* [10].

A. Gas Lasers [10, 26, 27]
   - One of the first lasers developed was the *helium-neon gas laser,* which has a visible red colour emission.
   - The most common gas in dental laser is *carbon dioxide*, which contains a gas mixture of carbon dioxide, helium, and nitrogen. Helium is not directly involved in the lasing process, whilst nitrogen interacts with the excitation process and ultimately transfers that energy to the carbon dioxide molecules.
   - Another gaseous laser is the *argon-ion instrument*. This noble gas when excited generates several radiant emissions, the most common being a visible blue and blue-green beam of collimated light. The physical demands of power and cooling have rendered this laser to a very limited application in dentistry.

B. Solid-State Crystal Lasers [10, 26, 28] The host material is composed of:
   - Yttrium aluminium garnet (YAG)
   - Yttrium aluminium perovskite (YAP), or
   - Yttrium scandium gallium garnet (YSGG)
   - Any of these can then be doped with ions of neodymium, erbium, and chromium. The resulting designation would be written as Nd:YAG, for example, which would be a neodymium-doped yttrium aluminium garnet crystal.

C. Semiconductor Dental Lasers [8-10, 26] A semiconductor laser utilizes the basic positive-negative (p-n) junction of everyday electronic circuits—the diode: that is, a two-pole oppositely charged wafer. The flow of negatively charged electrons into the positively charged holes diffuses across the junction. The lasing action takes place between the charged layers, called the depletion region. This small rectangle will emit coherent and monochromatic light, but collimation must be performed by an external lens. Current diode lasers consist of various atomic elements in binary, ternary, or quaternary forms arranged in a wafer-like structure. Examples would be:

1. Gallium arsenide (GaAs)
2. Aluminium gallium arsenide (AlGaAs)
3. Indium gallium arsenide (InGaAs), and
4. Indium gallium arsenide phosphate (InGaAsP)

These elements provide a checker board-like crystalline structure to allow lasing to occur; the usual silicon-based semiconductor is not used because of its symmetry. The single diode wafer just described is then arranged in a linear array for cooling, and the number of wafers determines the power output.

3.1.1. Working of an LED/p-n Junction [10]

The band structures of insulators and semiconductors are qualitatively similar. Normally there exists in both insulators and semiconductors a filled energy band (referred to as the valence band) separated from the next higher band (referred to as the conduction band) by an energy gap. For a semiconductor, the energy gap is usually smaller, about 1 electron volt. In general, the gap in insulators is at least several electron volts; overcoming this large energy gap to promote sufficient numbers of electrons to the conduction band cannot be achieved with an applied field or by thermal excitation. Therefore, there is high resistance to changing the total electron momentum and allowing the electrons to move as they would in a conductor. In a semiconductor, the valence band is full at very low temperatures (close to 0 K), but when the temperature increases, electrons acquire sufficient thermal energy to be promoted to the conduction band, which was empty initially. This effect creates the so-called "holes" in the valence band, which correspond to the "vacancies" left by the electrons that leave for the conduction band.

These holes can generate an electric current when an external electric field is applied because they represent the absence of negative charges. Conductivity of a material depends on the number of electrons that can be transferred to the conduction band and therefore are "free" to move within the crystalline arrangement. The number of electrons in the conduction band changes with temperature. Pure semiconductors are called "intrinsic," and because of their temperature dependence, they are not used in the manufacture of electrical devices (a device that only worked under a specific range of temperature would have limited utility). To use semiconductor materials, manufacturers usually use a technique called "doping," which means modifying the conductivity of a material by incorporating "impurities." This enables tighter control of the conduction conditions and allows different electronic devices to be made using the semiconductor. In the absence of an external electric field, the band gap is large enough for these semiconductors to act as insulators, but when an external field is applied, the balance of energy changes, and the electrons and holes acquire some degree of freedom. In this way, the behaviour of semiconductors can be controlled. Doped materials are usually called "extrinsic" materials. LEDs are made from two types of extrinsic material. The characteristics of the semiconductor will change depending on the impurities added. If impurities that can donate electrons are added, an "n-type" semiconductor ("n" for negative) is formed. These are usually made by introducing atoms with five electrons in their valence band, with the fifth electron weakly bound; consequently, these electrons are free to move around the crystal. Impurities in n-type materials are called donator atoms. The other kind of material is called a "p-type" semiconductor ("p" for positive), which is made by the addition of impurities that have only three valence electrons. In this case, the number of electrons is insufficient to make covalent bonds, creating holes in the crystalline array. Impurities with incomplete covalent bonds are called acceptor atoms. The "p–n" junction is at the base of the LED.

Table 1. Currently, available visible spectrum dental lasers

Type of Laser	Active Medium	Wavelength
Semiconductor diode, visible blue	Indium Gallium Nitride	445 nm
KTP solid state, visible light emission	Neodymium doped Yttrium Aluminium Garnet and Potassium Titanyl Phosphate	532 nm
Low-level lasers, visible red light emission, semiconductor or gas lasers	Variations of Gallium Arsenide or Indium Gallium Arsenide Phosphorus diodes or Helium-Neon gas	600-670 nm 632 nm

Table 2. Currently, available invisible infrared dental lasers

Type of Laser	Active Medium	Wavelength
Low-level lasers, (invisible) near infra-red	Variations in Aluminium Gallium Arsenide diode	800-900 nm
Semiconductor diode, near infrared	Aluminium Gallium Arsenide	800-830 nm
Semiconductor diode, near infrared	Aluminium/Indium Gallium Arsenide	940 nm
Semiconductor diode, near infrared	Indium Gallium Arsenide	980 nm
Semiconductor diode, near infrared	Indium Gallium Arsenide Phosphorus	1064 nm
Solid-state, near-infrared	Neodymium doped Yttrium Aluminium Garnet	1064 nm
Solid-state, near infrared	Neodymium doped Yttrium Aluminium Perovskite	1340 nm
Solid-state, mid-infrared	Erbium, Chromium doped Yttrium Scandium Gallium Garnet	2780 nm
Solid-state, mid-infrared	Erbium doped Yttrium Aluminium Garnet	2940 nm
Gas, far-infrared	Carbon dioxide laser with an active medium of isotopic gas	9300 nm
Gas, far-infrared	Carbon dioxide laser with an active medium of a mixture of gases	10,600 nm

The junction between a p-material and an n-material forms a semiconductor diode. The electrons in the "n" side move to the junction and will be projected into the "p" side to produce a high electron concentration in the conduction band, which is larger than when in thermal equilibrium. The same happens on the other side, with the holes. When an electron combines with a hole, energy is released, a fraction as thermal energy and another as a photon. When an external field is applied to the junction, the electrons and holes have sufficient energy to recombine and eventually emit a photon.

3.1.2. Pumping Mechanism

Surrounding this optical cavity with its active medium is an excitation source, known as the pumping mechanism. Pumping is used to transfer energy into the optical cavity, and that energy must be of sufficient quantity and duration so that the occupation of a higher energy level exceeds that of a lower level. This condition is called a *population inversion,* and it allows amplification to occur. Although the above-described process occurs rapidly, it still takes some time. Most lasers are described as three-level or four-level. A three-level system describes the basic concept: level one would be the stable, ground state, sometimes designated as energy level zero, a pumped level (energy level 2), and a lasing level (energy level.) Despite rapid decay from level 2, with enough pumped energy, there will be a population inversion between levels 1 and 2. A four-level system is similar, with the pumped level designated as 3, the upper lasing level as 2, and the lower lasing level as 1. The difference between these two lasing levels will aid in producing a population inversion. Certain active media operate as either three- or four-level systems [10, 29].

In the laser industry, there are a wide variety of pumping mechanisms. The pumping of dental lasers is usually performed with [25]:

1. Optical devices—high-power lamps or lasers
2. Electricity—either with direct current mains or with electronic modulation of alternating current.

Currently, diode lasers are electronically pumped; solid-state crystal lasers use high-powered strobes (flashlamps), and carbon dioxide lasers can be operated with AC or DC or radio frequency (RF) pumping methods.

3. As a variation in pumping, one form of carbon dioxide technology uses very high-pressure gas and many electrodes along the length of the gas tube. This is known as a transversely excited atmosphere (TEA) laser.

3.1.3. Optical Resonator

The resonator, sometimes known as the optical cavity or optical resonator, is the laser component surrounding the active medium. In most lasers, there are two mirrors one at each end of the optical cavity, placed parallel to each other, or in the case of a semiconductor, either a cleaved and polished surface exists at the end of the wafer or there is a reflection within the wafer. In all cases, these mirrored surfaces then produce constructive interference of the waves: that is, the incident wave and the reflected wave can superimpose on each other, producing an increase in their combined amplitude. Clearly, some waves will not combine and will soon lose their intensity, but others will continue to be amplified in this resonator. With the mirror system, this continued effect will help to collimate the developing beam. In a diode, laser collimation occurs externally [8, 10, 29].

3.2. Laser Delivery Systems [10]

Laser energy should be delivered to the site of interest precisely and ergonomically.

1. An optical fiber assembly
2. A hollow waveguide assembly
3. An articulated arm delivery system

3.2.1. Optical Fibre [10-12]

An optical glass fibre is usually made of quartz-silica. This glass core conducts the laser beam along its length. A thin polyamide coating surrounds the core to contain the light, and a pliable thicker jacket covers both, to protect the integrity of the system. A specific connector couples the fibre to the laser instrument; a hand piece and tip are added to the operative end.

3.2.2. Hollow Waveguide [10-12]

A hollow waveguide is a jacketed flexible tube. The internal surface has a reflective coating like silver iodide to allow the beam's transmission. A series of protective jackets complete the system. The waveguide is connected to the emission port on the laser, and a hand piece and optional tip are connected to the operative end.

3.2.3. Articulated Arm [10-12]

An articulated arm consists of a series of reflective hollow tubes with pivoting internally mirrored joints along its length. The arm has a counterweight to provide ease in movement. The laser emission port is coupled with the first tube, and a hand piece and optional tip are added to the operative end of the distal tube.

1. Shorter wavelength instruments, such as KTP, diode, and Nd:YAG lasers, have small, flexible fibre-optic systems with bare glass fibres or disposable tips that deliver the laser energy to the target tissue.
2. A few low-powered diode lasers are offered as handheld units with disposable glass tips.

3. Erbium devices are constructed with more rigid glass fibres, semi-flexible hollow waveguides, or articulated arms.
4. Carbon dioxide lasers use waveguides or articulated arms.
5. Some of the erbium systems employ small quartz or sapphire tips, and carbon dioxide instruments employ metal cylinders that are attached to the hand piece. All of the tips are used for contact with the target tissue, although they can direct the beam toward the tissue when not directly touching it. Other lasers in these wavelengths use tip-less (and therefore non-contact) delivery systems. In addition, some procedures demand that a clinician not directly contact the tissue.
6. In addition, the erbium lasers and the 9.3-micron carbon dioxide laser employ a water spray for cooling hard tissue.

Chapter 4

The Laser Beam

4.1. Monochromaticity or Near Monochromaticity

Laser beams are monochromatic, indicative of their composition with photons, all having the same wavelength (Figure 2). This attribute is dependent on the frequency and energy of the photon, indicating the precise electronic transitions generating those photons. Perfectly monochromatic light is a misnomer. However, laser light is significantly more monochromatic than the light from other commonly used sources. A consequence of monochromaticity is effective excitation with less power consumption. To elaborate, a given electron transition in a given medium will be more resourceful if the utilized photon has energy equivalent to or nearly equivalent to the transition energy because otherwise an enormous quantity of energy is exhausted in generating photons that are not used for the desired transition [10, 25, 29, 30]

4.2. Coherence

The photons within a laser beam are coherent, in that the waves are all in phase (their peaks and valleys line up) in terms of both space and time (Figure 2). There are two types of coherence: temporal and spatial. *Temporal coherence*, as explained by the Michelson interferometer arrangement, refers to how long in time, light waves remain in phase. *Spatial coherence*, as elucidated by Young's double-hole experiment, measures the area over which light is coherent [10].

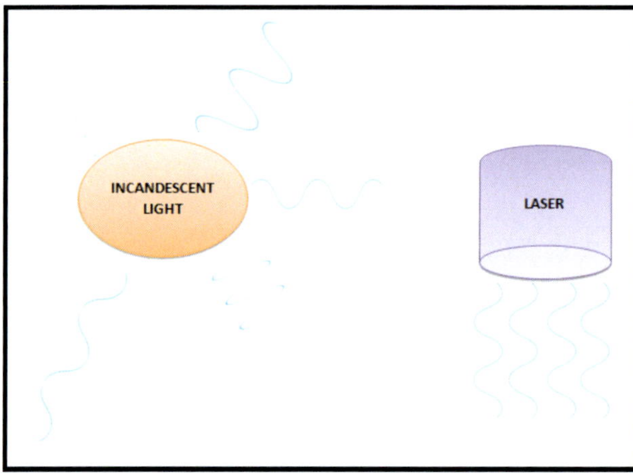

Figure 2. Incandescent light (divergent, incoherent, polychromatic) versus laser light (collimated, coherent, monochromatic).

4.3. Collimated with Directionality

All photons in a laser beam are parallel to each other. Hence, a laser beam is collimated (Figure 2). The importance lies in a minimally distorted propagation for exceedingly long distances and generation of a high-energy density congregated into a small volume. Directionality refers to the propagation of laser beam unidirectionally, with only a narrow cone of divergence. Consequently, as all output photons in the beam deviate minimally from the beam axis and travel mostly in the same direction, laser light may be many times more efficient when compared to a usual light source in terms of power output. Beam divergence depends on the nature of the resonator, the width of the emitting area, and diffraction, with the theoretical lower limit on beam divergence, addressed as the *diffraction limit* [4, 10, 30].

4.4. Radiance

Radiance refers to the power emitted per unit surface area of source per unit solid angle. Owing to the property of directionality, the lasers have large radiance. High radiance indicates that the beam can be propagated to large distances without much loss of intensity [4].

4.5. Focusability

The small laser beam divergence implies that lasers can be focused on small spot sizes. Owed to its focusability, laser light can be efficiently coupled to thin optical fibres rendering endoscopically guided applications [4].

4.6. Spectral Coverage

Lasers are available from vacuum ultraviolet to millimetre spectral region. Still shorter frequencies have been generated using non-linear optical techniques [4].

4.7. Gating and Pulsing

Surgical lasers have a mechanical shutter positioning mechanism. A timing circuit controls the opening and closing of the circuit. According to timing, they can be continuous, gated, and pulsed (Figure 3) [3].

Compared with continuous lasers, intermittent laser energy pulses accomplish a reduction in collateral damage, in between cooling of the target, as well as an increase in the power per pulse. The 2 types of pulsed laser delivery include the use of a mechanical shutter (pulsed laser) or a resonance chamber (Q switch and pico lasers) [1]. An elementary distinction between these deliveries is that Q-switched and pico lasers can have significantly higher peak energies than the pulsed and continuous lasers [25].

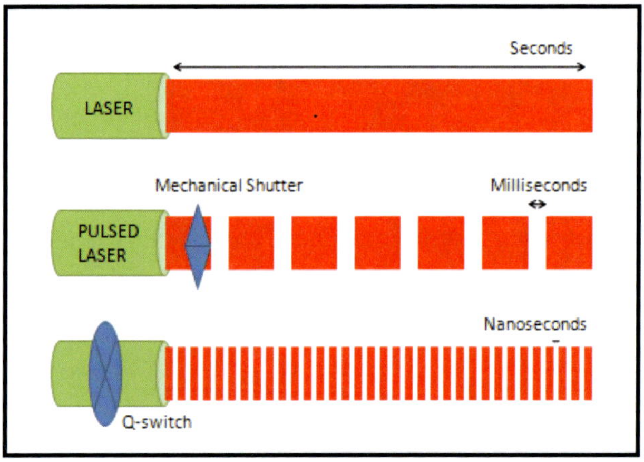

Figure 3. Continuous versus intermittent pulse patterns.

4.8. Beam Profile

Beam profile refers to the cross-section of the beam. There can be two beam profiles for a laser: *Fundamental or Gaussian beam profile* (greater concentration of photons in beam core with diminution of light intensity at edges) and *Donut profile* (cold spot in centre) [30, 31].

4.9. Spot Geometry

The projection of the beam on the target is called a 'spot'. The diameter of this spot is called a spot size. Spot size is reduced with a progressive increase in depth [10, 30].

4.10. Focal Length and Focal Point

The lens incorporated resolves the focal length. There are three terminologies used in this reference, i.e., focused, defocused mode, and pre-focused mode (Figure 4) [30, 31].

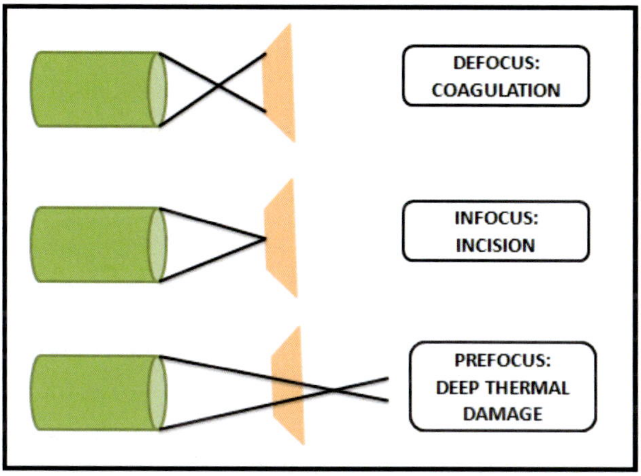

Figure 4. Focusing modes of the laser beam.

Chapter 5

Laser-Tissue Interactions

The various phenomena encompassing laser–tissue interactions form the foundation of the expediency of predictable usage of laser photonics as an accessory to clinical oro-dental therapy.

5.1. Reflection and Refraction

Reflection ensues when electromagnetic radiation rebounds back from the surface on which it was focused. A physical interfacial separation between two materials, differing in their refractive indexes, forms a reflecting surface. Specular reflection occurs when a smooth surface is encountered, wherein it is implicit that any surface/interfacial imperfections are small compared to the wavelength of the incident radiation. Diffuse reflections, a commonplace with biological tissues, occur when surface imperfections are equal to or greater than the wavelength of the incident radiation [10, 11]. Refraction occurs when a reflective interface partitions two media with diverse refractive indexes. This circumstance is the outcome of variations in the incident light velocity. Both the above phenomena reckon on additional parameters, namely angle of incidence and polarization of the radiation. The Fresnel's law expounds the association between reflection and refraction [10].

5.2. Absorption and Transmission [10-12]

The phenomenon of absorption occurs when the electromagnetic radiation neither rebounds from the incident surface nor propagates in the tissue. *Absorbance* is measured as the ratio of the intensity of radiation absorbed to intensity of radiation incident which banks on parameters namely atomic and molecular electronic constitution, radiation wavelength, absorber(s) thickness and concentration, and temperature of the internal milieu. For a transparent medium, the energy that is incident is equiponderant to that exiting the medium, owing to the complete passage of all incident light without absorption. The incident radiation energy is attenuated close to null when an opaque medium is considered. The above-stated properties are chiefly dependent upon the incident light wavelength. A fraction of incident radiation is converted into heat or kinetic energy [10-12]. Macromolecular constituents, namely proteins and pigments along with water, are principally accountable for all biological tissue absorption. The *therapeutic window* (600 nm and 1200 nm), frequently relied on for LLLT, is absorbed more deeply into biological tissues [4, 25]. The relationship between absorber thickness and absorption and concentration and absorption is dissertated by *Beer–Lambert's law*[10] ($I_{(x)} = I_0 e^{-\alpha x}$) *Beer's law* ($I_{(z)} = I_0 e^{-k'CZ}$) respectively, where z = optical axis, $I_{(z)}$ = light intensity at distance z, I_0 = initial intensity of light, α = absorption coefficient of the medium, c = concentration of absorbers, and k' = internal parameters.

5.3. Scattering [4, 10, 11]

Resonance, as a phenomenon, manifests when the frequency of the incident wave and the natural frequency of vibration of free particles of the tissue irradiated are co-incident or equal. On the contrary, when the frequency of incident light does not match the natural frequency of the vibration of particles, scattering manifests. While resonance is attended by sizeable absorption, scattering can be measured as the fundamental basis of the dispersion. When the incident and scattered photons are equi-energetic, an *elastic scattering* is observed while *inelastic scattering* is seen otherwise [10, 11]. *Rayleigh scattering,* a variant of elastic scattering, mandates that the particles scattered must be smaller compared to the wavelength of the incident radiation. Rayleigh´s law (~1/λ4) gives the scattered intensity and refractive index. When the scattered particles are dimensionally equivalent to the incident wavelength, *Mie scattering* occurs, which shows feeble reliance on incident wavelength. A probability function p(θ) of a photon to be scattered at an angle θ is necessitated, as neither Rayleigh nor Mie scattering suffices the explanation of scattering in biological mediums. If a dependency between probability function and angle θ is established, the scattering is *anisotropic*, otherwise, it is isotropic scattering [4, 10].

The laser-tissue interactions have been pictorially summarized in Figure 5.

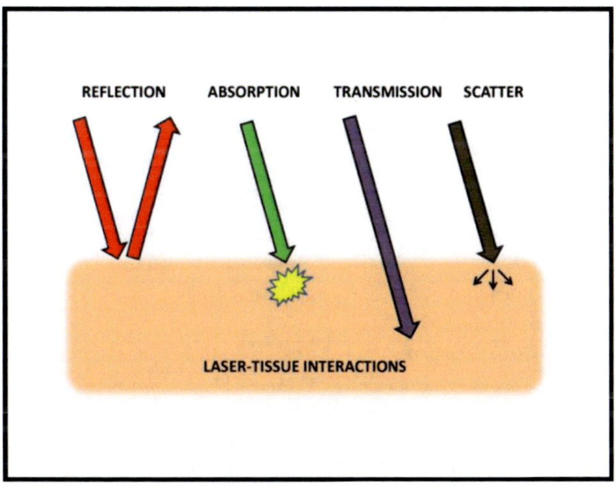

Figure 5. Pictorial representation of various laser-tissue interactions.

5.4. TISSUE EFFECTS OF LASER IRRADIATION

Parameters that determine the type of laser-tissue interaction (Figure 6) include its wavelength, power density, and exposure duration.

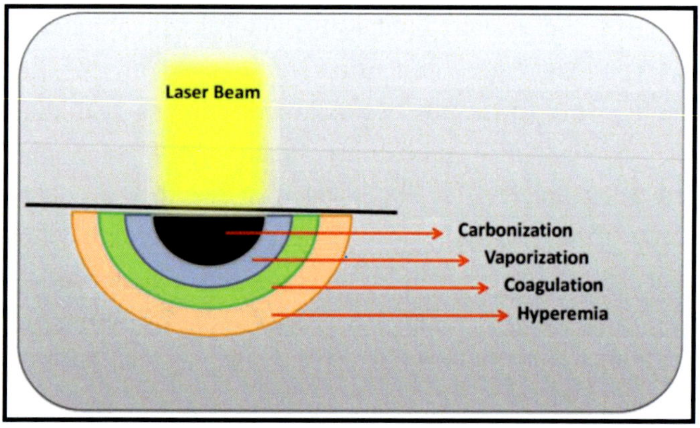

Figure 6. Tissue effects of laser irradiation.

Table 3. Effects of temperature on soft tissues [10]

Temperature (°C)	Primary effect	Secondary effect
37	None	None
42	Tissue heating	Damage to some chemical bonds; alterations in cell membranes; necrosis of small areas
50	Diminution of enzymatic activity	Cellular ablation
60	Tissue denaturation	Tissue coagulation, necrosis, bleaching
80	Changes in membrane permeability	Chemical bond destruction
100	Cutting, vaporization	Thermal decomposition
150	Carbonization	Darkening of the tissue (avoided by coolant usage)
400	Melting	Fast incision

On absorption of radiant energy by tissue, the fundamental responses encompass: (a) Photochemical interaction, (b) Photothermal interaction, (c) Photomechanical interaction, and (d) Photoelectrical interaction.

- Photochemical interaction appends biostimulation, photodynamic therapy, and tissue fluorescence. The indispensable fundamental governing this process is the interaction of specific wavelengths with endogenous chromospheres or with artificial dyes/photo sensitizers to encourage in-vivo biologic reactions facilitating diagnostic and therapeutic purposes [30, 32]
- Photothermal interaction encompasses photoablation (tissue removal by vaporization/superheating), coagulation, hemostasis, photopyrolysis (tissue burning). Selective photothermolysis, pioneered by Anderson and Parrish [34] explicates the principles for clinical utility of photothermal lasers. Selective photothermolysis relies on the following primaries: 1) The wavelength of laser light chosen must be selective and appropriate for the target tissue [25, 34] 2) The target tissue must be destroyed without damaging the surrounding tissues. 3) The pulse width or duration of the laser pulse must be within the thermal relaxation time of the treated tissues. Thermal relaxation time is the amount of time it takes to transfer two-thirds of the resultant heat to the surrounding tissues. 4) Varying the pulse width, fluence, and spot size will have varying effects from ablation, ranging from vaporization of skin during CO_2 laser resurfacing to the consequent inflammatory response to mild thermal injury as with photorejuvenation [34].
- Photomechanical interaction includes photo disruption or photo disassociation utilized for cavity preparation, caries, and restorative materials removal [30, 32]
- Photoelectric interactions entail photoplasmolysis, which is the removal of tissue by formation by electrically charged ions contemporarily used for nerve repair and regeneration [30, 33]

Table 4. Effects of temperature on dental hard tissues [10]

Temperature (°C)	Primary effect
100-140	Evaporation of water
250–400	Oxidation and pyrolysis of organic compounds
100–650	Conversion of phosphate to pyrophosphates
500–900	Carbon oxidation of organic matrix and decomposition of carbonate of inorganic phase
700–850	Total decomposition of carbonate of inorganic phase
1000–1100	Formation of tricalcium phosphates, tetracalcium phosphate, and bruxite
1280	Melting of enamel and natural hydroxyapatite

Chapter 6

LASER TERMINOLOGIES AND DOSIMETRY

The laser equipment has a unique and unalterable photon energy emission attributed to its wavelength [4, 11, 30].

The clinician, however, can adjust various parameters of that emission (Table 5) from both the control panel and the hand piece's position on the target tissue, to acquire preferred effects as demonstrated in Figures 7, 8, 9, 10.

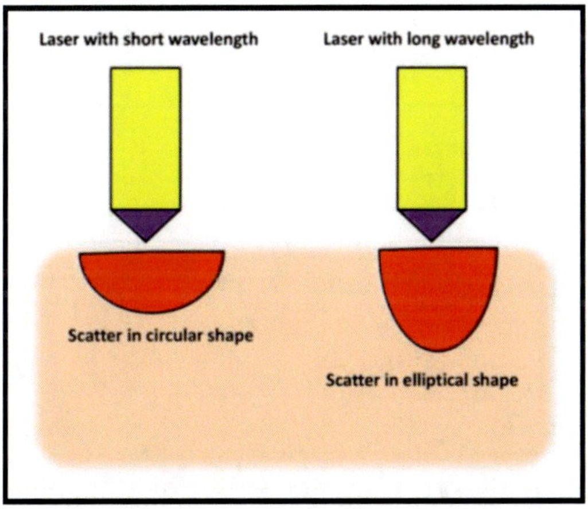

Figure 7. Shape of the light profile in illuminated or irradiated tissue.

Table 5. Summary of laser terminologies and dosimetry

Term	Definition	Unit
Energy	The ability to do work	J (joule) or mJ (mill joule)
Fluence	Energy per area, energy density	J/cm^2
Power	Work performed over time	W (watt)
Power density	Power per area	W/cm2
Beam size	The area of the projected laser beam on the tissue	(Usually measured in microns or millimetres)

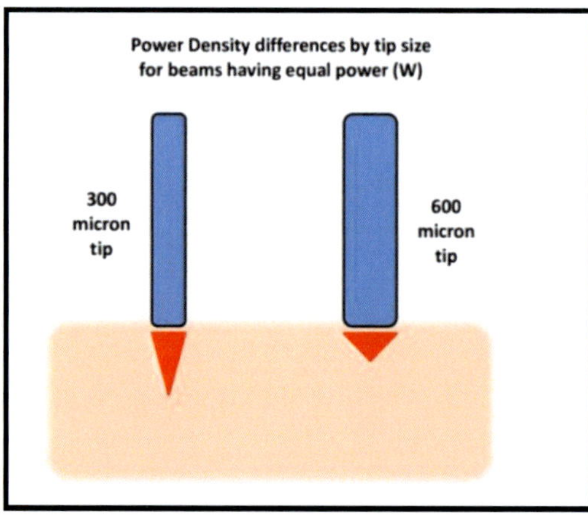

Figure 8. Difference between power density areas using a 300-micron tip/beam size and a 600-micron tip/beam size. The smaller fibre has a larger area of interaction because of the larger power density.

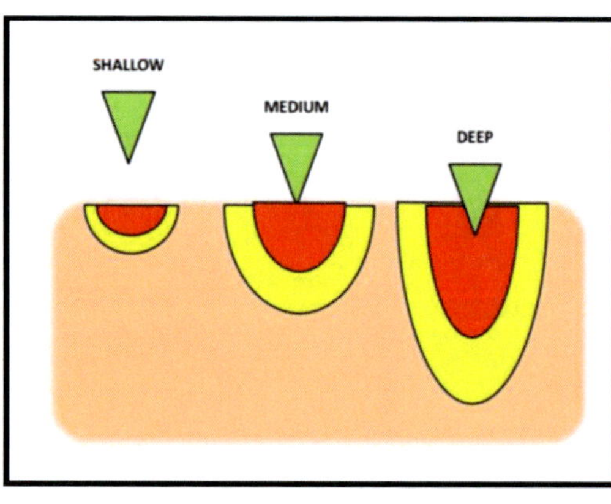

Figure 9. Three modes of laser treatment.

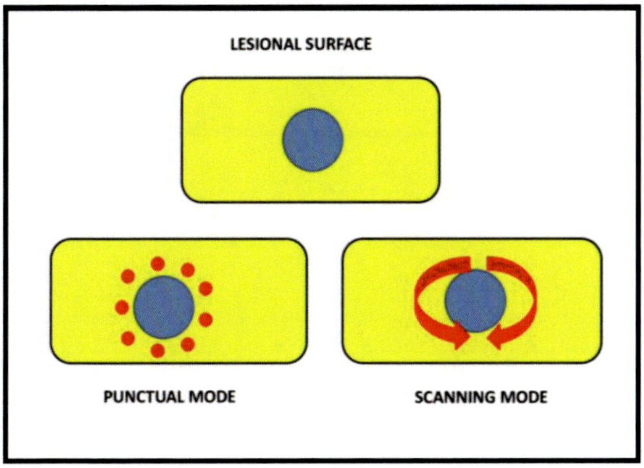

Figure 10. Scanning and punctual irradiation modes.

Chapter 7

LASER HAZARDS AND CONTRAINDICATIONS

There are various laser hazards that can be classified in various categories (Table 6, 7), which could be harmful to individuals and can lead to potential damage to the human body.

Table 6. According to Walsh, based on potential hazards, the laser can be classified into I, II, IIIA, IIIB, and IV [35]

Class	Risk	Example
I	Fully enclosed system	Nd:YAG laser welding system used in the dental laboratory
II	Visible low power lasers protected by blink reflex	A Visible red aiming beam of a surgical laser
III a	Visible laser above 1 mill watt	No dental examples
III b	High power laser units that may or may not be visible. Direct viewing is hazardous to the eyes.	Low power diode lasers used for biostimulation
IV	Damage to eyes and skin possible. Direct or indirect viewing is hazardous to the eyes.	All lasers used for oral surgery, whitening, and cavity preparation

Dental lasers belong to category IV that is the most hazardous of all the lasers. According to Miserendino et al. (1995), the types of hazards that can be encountered within the clinical practice of dentistry are grouped as follows:

- Ocular injury
- Tissue damage
- Respiratory hazards
- Fire and explosion
- Electrical shock

Table 7. Classification according to American National Standards Institute (ANSI), Occupational Safety, and Health Administration (OHSA) [35]

Class	Description
I	Low power lasers that are safe to view
II a	Low power visible lasers that are hazardous only when viewed directly for a longer time (>1000s)
II b	Low power visible lasers are hazardous when viewed for >0.25 s
III a	Medium power lasers or systems that are normally not hazardous if viewed for <0.25 s without magnifying optics
III b	Medium power lasers (0.5 W maximum) that can be hazardous when viewed directly
IV	High power lasers (>0.5 W) that produce ocular, skin, and fire hazards

7.1. Ocular Injury/Hazards

Table 8. Types of damage sustained by non-protected ocular structures exposed to laser beams of varying incident wavelengths [11]

Incident laser wavelength	Pathological effect
315–400 nm (UV-A)	Photochemical cataract (clouding of the eye lens)
400–780 nm (visible)	Photochemical damage to the retina, retinal burn
780–1400 nm (near-IR)	Cataract, retinal burn
1.4–3.0 μm (mid-IR)	Aqueous flare (protein in the aqueous humor), cataract, corneal burn
3.0 μm–10.6 μm (far IR)	Corneal burn

Potential injury to the eye can occur by direct emission either from the laser or by the reflection from a specular (mirror-like) surface (Table 8). According to Miserendino et al. (1995), dental instruments have been capable of producing reflections that may result in tissue damage to both operator and patient [35]. Sosis recommended the use of carbonized or non-reflective instruments during laser treatment by some authorities [36].

7.2. TISSUE HAZARDS

The tissue hazards could be of two types of reactions, thermal interactions, and non-thermal interactions.

1. Thermal interactions: Laser-induced damage to the skin and other non-target tissue can result from the thermal interaction of energy with tissue proteins. Temperature elevations of 21°C or above normal body temperature (37°C) can lead to cell destruction by denaturation of cellular enzymes and structural proteins. Exposures of one s or more than that can lead to vascular perfusion and thermal diffusion of heat energy within the tissue. In the case of wavelength being more than 400 nm, there could be thermal coagulation necrosis [35, 36].
2. Non-thermal tissue interaction: It induces tissue injury by photochemical and photoacoustic mechanisms. This type of interaction is most likely to occur with single or repetitive pulses of very short duration (<10 s). It can cause radiant exposures within the ultraviolet spectrum, such as those with excimer lasers.

Hence, laser-induced tissue injury is primarily dependent on the extent of absorption of radiation by tissue. However, it is important to know that there are certain factors that affect the extent of laser-tissue interaction such as [11, 35]:

1. The relative amount of absorption, transmission, and scatter of the particular wavelength, (2) The pulse duration and pulse repetition rate,
2. The level of radiant exposure (energy density or exposure dose), and
3. The relative degree of vascularity of the tissue.

During ablation of oral tissue with the carbon dioxide laser, a carbonized layer of tissue residue, or char layer forms on the surface. This carbon material is a strong absorber of laser wavelength. It acts as a heat sink that transfers energy to surrounding tissues.

The mode of delivery of laser wavelength is an important factor to induce the nature of the interaction. Lasers such as neodymium: yttrium-aluminum-garnet (Nd:YAG) with a non-contact system will produce different effects with more penetration into deeper structures as compared to that of a contact tip laser scalpel.

7.3. Environmental Hazards

Miserendino et al. (1995) described another type of hazard, which involves the inhalation of airborne biohazards materials that is released during the surgical procedure of laser. These types of hazards are sometimes referred to as non-beam hazards [35, 36], as they do not cause tissue injury from direct exposure to the laser beam. Inhaled air-borne contaminants can be emitted in the form of smoke or plume generated through the thermal interaction of surgical lasers. Most surgical lasers used in dentistry are capable of smoke generation, toxic gases, and chemicals, which are more common hazards in dental research (e.g., excimer laser). During ablation or incision of oral soft tissue, cellular products are vaporized due to the rapid heating of the liquid components in the tissue. In the process, extremely small fragments of carbonized, partially carbonized, and relatively intact tissue elements are violently projected into the area, creating airborne contaminants that are observed clinically as smoke or what is commonly called the laser plume [11].

The extent of plume generation depends on the absorption of various wavelengths by the target tissue. The greatest producers of smoke are the carbon dioxide and erbium lasers, and then, Nd:YAG laser. Carbon dioxide and erbium: yttrium-aluminum-garnet (Er:YAG) lasers have high-coefficient absorption because of the high-water content of oral tissue.

7.4. Combustion Hazards

Flammable solids, liquids, and gases used within the surgical setting can be easily ignited if exposed to the laser beam. Here, nitrous oxide is generally considered as non-flammable material but will support combustion [35, 37].

7.5. Electrical Hazards

According to Miserendino et al. (1995), class IV lasers need high currents and high voltage power supplies. They sub grouped electrical hazards of lasers as electrical shock hazards, electrical fire hazards, or explosion hazards. The laser system may get exposed to conductive liquids that may contribute to an electrical hazard [36].

7.6. Contraindications of Lasers

The contraindications can be divided into the following three principal groups [38]:

1. Justified
2. Doubtful under certain conditions; and
3. Erroneous

7.6.1. Justified Contraindications

1. Noninvasive laser therapy is unambiguously contraindicated in malignant diseases with respect to the experimentally demonstrated biostimulating effect [39]
2. In suspected or diagnosed cases of Thyroid gland disease, laser application in this region should be used with maximum caution [40]
3. Certain authors also consider epilepsy as a serious contraindication of noninvasive laser therapy. In spite of the fact that the cause of the induction of a seizure in the therapeutic laser application is not clear, it is assumed that an epileptic seizure can possibly be induced when selecting a certain frequency of the pulsed beam, which is, however, different for each patient [40]
4. Direct irradiation of the retina is a generally recognized contraindication [40]
5. In the therapeutic laser application, we also avoid the irradiation of the abdominal and of course also the intravaginal region in gravid women [41]
6. Prior to starting the treatment with a therapeutic laser, it is necessary to be sure that the patient has not taken a drug or massage product and that he or she does not use cosmetic products containing photosensitizers (e.g., cosmetic self-tanning creams) [42]

7.6.2. Contraindications Doubtful Under Certain Conditions

- Certain authors consider the use of therapeutic lasers to be contraindicated in feverish conditions and infectious diseases. It is, however, always necessary to consider the particular health condition and aetiology of the disease itself [38]
- In the literature, there are recommendations that the laser should not be applied in patients with haematological diseases without specifying what diseases are considered. In this connection, haematological diseases include, on the one hand, mild hypochromic anaemia and, on the other hand, life-endangering myeloblastic leukaemia. Whereas the principles we specified above hold for the use of the therapeutic laser in malignant haematological diseases, it is useless to avoid this type of treatment, for example, in anaemia. Few authors have demonstrated that the laser therapy itself does not affect the period of life of blood cells, and there is no reason for avoiding its application in any field except for irradiating hemopoietic bone marrow [38]
- Caution is also necessary when applying the therapeutic laser in patients with considerable blood loss due to the laser therapy vasodilating effect [43]
- The analgesic effect of noninvasive laser therapy is given by reducing the sensitivity of proprioreceptors in the skin. Thus, caution is necessary in neuropathies, since the application of a therapeutic laser will reduce the existing minimum sensitivity with a danger of damaging the given region, for example, by sun exposure [44]
- The application of the therapeutic laser in the region of gonads also cannot be considered contraindicated. It should only be performed at specialized working sites with sufficient experience with this type of treatment. At lower energy densities (up to 1.3 J/cm^2), the laser exerts a stimulating effect on germ cells of men; however, possibilities of mutations cannot be precluded when

increasing the energy density. No negative effect of noninvasive laser therapy was observed in women, even in the case of the intravaginal application [38]

7.6.3. Erroneous Contraindications

- Use of therapeutic laser in persons with cardio-stimulators. In the case of the correctness of this contraindication, this would mean that in patients with an implanted cardio-stimulator, the x-ray examination and exposure of the skin to solar radiation is also contraindicated [38].
- Further doubtful contraindications are exhaustion, cachexia, or dependence on alcohol and/or drugs. This contraindication also cannot be considered correct [38]
- The local application of the therapeutic laser in certain indications (non-healing wounds after administration of drugs) is even beneficial for a patient and, with respect to minimum side effects, it is less aggressive to the patient than pharmacotherapy [38]
- Fear of possible damage to the epiphyseal slots in children in the case of the application of therapeutic laser is baseless [38,41]

Chapter 8

LASER SAFETY

Safety is an important and integral part of any device or instrument before use. When we evaluate a product such as a dental laser for its use in patients, we must consider its safety before its use along with its effectiveness and efficacy. Here, the risk-benefit ratio should be small, and the device should be more beneficial to the patients [11, 36].

According to Piccione, three factors are important to laser safety [45]:

1. The manufacturing process of the instrument.
2. Proper operation of the device.
3. The personal protection of the surgical team and the patient.

For the safety of a laser device and its practice, regulatory agencies play an important role. The United States has four major organizations and agencies, which form regulations and rules for the safety of laser systems. They are the ANSI; the Food and Drug Administration (FDA) and its regulatory bureau, the CDRH, and the OHSA [35].

8.1. Laser Device Hardware Safety Measures [11, 35, 36]

1. Locked unit panels to prevent unauthorized access to internal machinery.
2. Control panel to ensure correct emission parameters.
3. Emission port shutters to prevent laser emission until the correct delivery system is attached.
4. Covered foot switch, to prevent accidental operation.
5. Remote interlocks to govern against accidental access to the operatory by unauthorized and non-protected personnel.
6. Casters, if present, must be lockable.

8.2. Safety Measures During Laser Use [11]

1. Key or password protection. When disabled (key or code removed), the laser cannot be operated.
2. Laser software diagnostics and error messages.
3. Display of parameters.
4. Audible or visual signs of laser emission – recommended as an area control for Class IIIB laser operation. Such a warning system is mandatory for Class IV lasers.
5. Specific standby and laser emission modes.
6. Time-lapsed default to standby mode Class IV lasers requires a permanently attached beam stop or attenuator, which can reduce the output emission to a level at or below the appropriate MPE level when the laser system is on "standby."
7. Emergency "stop" button.

For all operators using lasers within the delivery of dental care, safety protocol may be seen within four areas [11, 46]:

1. The physical dimensions of the care delivery area – the "controlled area" and "nominal ocular hazard zone". "Laser protection advisor" role.
2. The duties of the "laser safety officer" in determining and enforcing safety within the controlled area during delivery of dental care to patients.
3. Physical laser protection of the eyes, skin, and general sterility within the controlled area.
4. Local rules, record-keeping and adverse reaction protocols.
5. Adequate staff training.

8.3. Fire and Electrical Control Measures [46]

To avoid electrical hazards during laser operation, the floor of the operatory room should be kept dry. As we know, the laser generates heat; hence care should be taken to avoid the use of flammable or explosive liquids or gases in the operation theatre. Certain combustible materials can be ignited by exposure to the laser beam.

8.4. Laser Test Fire Procedure [11]

This is designed to allow all working components of the laser to be checked before attempting the clinical procedure on the patient and is performed by the LSO or the dentist.

1. Warning signs on the door/window, protection and interlocks employed, to prevent unauthorized access as though a laser procedure was being performed.
2. All personnel within the controlled area should wear appropriate eye protection before the laser device is switched on.

3. The laser delivery system is assembled and minimum operating parameters are chosen. The laser is directed away from the eyes and a suitable absorption medium should be used. The laser is fired within that medium so that the beam is attenuated. The use of an approved laser power meter allows the LSO to check the parameter display on the laser control panel and to check the value against the meter reading. Associated with this check is the opportunity with many laser units to use a calibration port on the laser as part of the set-up procedure.
4. For visible and near-infrared wavelengths, a suitable medium would be pigmented/dark articulating paper, and for longer mid- and far-infrared wavelengths (erbium family and carbon dioxide), the suitable medium should be water. The objectives of the laser test-fire are to check the following:
    a. Test the operational ability of the machine.
    b. Test cleavability of fibre (where appropriate).
    c. Demonstrate patency of delivery mechanism.
    d. Demonstrate patency of aiming beam/coaxial air/water.

8.5. Eye Protection During Laser Use [35, 36, 45]

1. A protocol to use is mandatory, including "patient on first – off last" as a maxim to represent the safety of the patient as paramount. With the patient considered first, each member of the clinical team within the controlled area would be obliged to similarly wear eye protection.
2. Glasses/goggles must cover the entire peri-orbital region, be free of any surface scratches or damage, and be fitted with suitable side panels to prevent diffuse laser beam entry.
3. Eyewear should be constructed of wavelength-specific material to attenuate the laser energy or to contain the energy within MPE values.

4. Glasses or goggles should be marked with the wavelength for which protection is given, either as a specific wavelength value or range of wavelengths within which protection may be afforded by the chosen eyewear. The level of protection is specifically expressed in terms of optical density (OD). This quantitative measurement represents the ability of the eyewear lens material to reduce laser energy of a specific wavelength to a safe level below the MPE. The OD value is measured as a log10 scale of laser beam attenuation and should be "5.0" or above for adequate protection.
5. Worldwide, the minimum information that must be present on protective eyewear (laser wavelength or a range of wavelengths that are covered by the material and OD value) may be further enhanced according to the nature of the eyewear, its specific intended use, and other factors pertinent to national, regional, or continental regulations. This additional information can be referenced against laser safety requirements (ANSI/IEC/EN) for individual laser clinicians, and laser protection advisors/laser safety officers may provide additional advice. Examples of supplemental eyewear data may include: "DIR" defines the emission mode of the laser for which the eyewear is intended. "D" signifies continuous-wave emission (CW), "I" pulsed mode, and "R" Q-switched mode. The significance of this is further enhanced in respect of "DIN": direct impact number – this is the ability of the eyewear material to attenuate direct laser beam energy within MPE limits. "L6A": a protective grade, which defines suitability for use of the protective eyewear within an intended clinical, industrial, or research condition. "CE" logo: "Conformité Européenne" will indicate a license approved for distribution and use within the countries of the European community. Manufacturer's identification mark
6. An increasing number of dental practitioners use loupes during clinical work, and such magnification may significantly increase the risk to the unprotected eye. For those procedures and laser

classes of risk to the eye when using loupes (laser Classes IM, II, IIM, IIIR, IIIB, and Class IV), the clinician must wear the appropriate protective insert or shield that is specific to the wavelength being used.

8.6. Control Measures for Airborne Contaminants [35, 46]

The airborne contaminants are smoke or vapour generated from the surgical site are known as laser plume. It is believed that exposure to carbon dioxide laser smoke can affect the respiratory system. Miserendino et al. (1995) stated that airborne contaminants could be controlled by ventilation, evacuation, or various methods of respiratory protection. They recommended evacuation of airborne contaminants as close as possible from the surgical point of origin. Sufficient suction in the surgical field should be maintained, especially in pathological conditions with the aetiology of viral infection, to limit the possibility of spreading the virus through laser plume. The evacuation system should be able to remove the smallest size of particles, and the filter in the system should be changed regularly as per the manufacturer's instruction to improve efficiency. Surgical staff must wear a mask during laser activation.

Chapter 9

Low Power Lasers and Their Applications

9.1. Introduction to Low Power Lasers

The names to identify and differentiate therapeutic lasers from surgical lasers include soft, cold, low-intensity laser therapy, LLLT, healing laser, non-thermal laser, therapeutic lasers, bioregulation laser, and biostimulation laser [47]. Therapeutic lasers are classified as class III medical devices, and surgical lasers are classified as class IV [48]. The use of LLLT has been documented in the literature for more than 30 years. Endre Mester in Budapest in the late 1960s pioneered the biostimulatory effect of low-level laser, which demonstrated an increase in collagen synthesis in skin wounds [49].

The photophysical–chemical actions of low power lasers are founded on whether their main interaction is with endogenous or exogenous photoacceptors: [10]

1. Photobiomodulation (known as laser therapy or LLLT) and
2. Photodynamic therapy (PDT), which depends on the interaction of the laser light with a photosensitizer that produces reactive oxygen species (ROS) upon irradiation with light, leading to

microbial reduction (in this case, named Antimicrobial Photodynamic Therapy – aPDT) or cell death. It is important to highlight that in PDT, the photosensitizer absorbs most of the laser light and biomodulation effects are minimal.

Several parameters characterize LLLT. These are as follows: [50]

1. Laser power: Ranges from 10–3 to 10–1 W
2. Wavelength: Ranges from 300 to 10,600 nm
3. Pulse rate: Range from 0 to 5000 Hz
4. Intensity: Ranging from 10–2 to 102 J/cm^2
5. Electromagnetic spectrum: Therapeutic lasers are within visible red to near-visible red ranging from 630 to 980 nm.

Table 9. Promising applications of LLLT [51]

Soft tissue applications	**Hard tissue applications**
Herpetic lesions	Temporomandibular disorders
Aphthous/traumatic ulcers	Orthodontic treatment
Post radiation mucositis	Dentinal hypersensitivity
Post extraction wound/socket healing	Bone remodelling
Trigeminal neuralgia	The stimulatory effect on root development
Periodontal disinfection	Implants
Post-surgical pain	
Gag reflex/nausea	
Sinusitis	
Edema	

9.2. Cellular Mechanisms of Photobiomodulation

The delivery of monochromatic and quasi-monochromatic photonic energy in the sub-ablative range (600–1000 nm) to biological tissues initiates and modulates various photobiological cellular responses that entail low-level light therapy (LLLT), otherwise referred to as phototherapy or photobiomodulation) [10, 11] The effectual tissue penetration of light is maximized within a so-called optical window in tissue (approx. 650 nm–1100 nm), consequent to which LLLT incorporates almost exclusively red and near-infrared light (600– 1100 nm). This overall phenomenon is governed by the first law of photobiology (Sutherland 2002), which affirms that for execution of the biological effect upon irradiation by low power visible light, the incident photons must undergo electronic absorption by molecular photoacceptors, or chromophores [52].

9.2.1. NO Hypothesis

The concentration of NO is up regulated primarily owing to macrophage activation. There occurs a consequent reversible inhibition in the activity of cytochrome c oxidase [54]. This is expounded by direct competition between NO and O2 for the reduced binuclear centre CuB/a^3 of cytochrome c oxidase. This may produce an increase in levels of the oxidized form of CuB. Owing to a weak coordinate binding, laser irradiation could reverse the partial inhibition of this catalytic center by NO, by photodissociating NO and thus increasing the O2-binding and respiration rate. An additional mechanism cited is the protective effect on cells against NO-induced cell death [10, 55].

9.2.2. Transient Local Heating Hypothesis

An ambient increase in local temperature of absorbing chromophores occurs upon excitation of its electronic states and release of a fraction of this excitation energy as heat.

This temperature escalation may induce structural-conformational alterations and prompt biochemical activity namely signalling of cellular pathways or secondary dark reactions [10, 52].

9.2.3. Mitochondrial Respiration and ATP

An augmentation for ATP, a universal driving biological fuel, may promote metabolism, in otherwise ailing or subdued cells. ATP has a dual role in being an energy currency as well as a paramount signalling molecule. Additionally, as a neurotransmitter, ATP is directly involved in a multitude of neuronal functions. Protective responses such as bone formation and cell proliferation are set off when ATP is elaborated by non-neuronal cells [10]. Cells of skin like keratinocytes and fibroblasts elaborate good amounts of ATP when exposed to heat or electric current [52, 53].

Cytochrome c oxidase (Cox) is a multi-component membrane protein that contains a binuclear copper centre (CuA) along with a heme binuclear centre (a3-CuB), both of which facilitate the transfer of electrons from water-soluble cytochrome c oxidase to oxygen. It is a terminal enzyme of the electron transport chain and plays a vital role in the bioenergetics of a cell. It was proposed that Cox is the primary photo acceptor for the red-NIR range in mammalian cells because absorption spectra obtained for Cox in different oxidation states were found to be very similar to the action spectra for biological responses to light. The absorption of photons by Cox leads to electronically excited states and consequently can lead to the quickening of electron transfer reactions. More electron transport necessarily causes increased production of ATP. The light-induced increase in ATP synthesis and increased proton gradient lead to increasing activity of the Na+/H+ and Ca2+/Na+ antiporters, and of all the ATP-driven carriers for ions, such as Na+/K+ ATPase and Ca2+ pumps. ATP is the substrate for adenylcyclase, and therefore the ATP level controls the level of cAMP. Both Ca2+and cAMP are very important second messengers [54].

9.2.4. Reactive Oxygen Species (ROS) and Gene Transcription

LLLT causes a reallocation in overall cell redox potential, favouring a trend of greater oxidation and increased ROS generation. The redox state of a cell controls cellular signalling pathways that control gene expression. Changes in redox state induce the activation of numerous intracellular signaling pathways, such as nucleic acid synthesis, protein synthesis, enzyme activation, and cell cycle progression. These cytosolic responses may induce transcriptional changes. Among them redox factor-1 (Ref-1)-dependent activator protein-1 (AP-1) (Fos and Jun), nuclear factor B (NFB), p53, activating transcription factor/cAMP-response element-binding protein (ATF/ CREB), hypoxia-inducible factor (HIF)-1 and HIF-like factor are the most important factors [53, 56].

9.2.5. Role in Gene Expression [54]

Table 10. The effects of LLL on gene expression [54]

Name of gene	Role	Change
Mitogen-activated protein kinase 11 (MAPK 11)	Proliferation	Up regulation
Breakpoint Cluster Region (BCR)	Proliferation	Up regulation
Serum response factor	Proliferation	Up regulation
Cullin 1	Prevent proliferation	Down regulation
Heat shock 70kd protein 1A Caspase 6 stress Induced phosphoprotein-1	Apoptosis	Down regulation
NADH dehydrogenase (ubiquinone) 1 beta, 2	Energy metabolism and respiratory chain	Up regulation
ATP syntheses	Energy metabolism and respiratory chain	Up regulation
Electron transfer flavoprotein, beta polypeptide	Energy metabolism and respiratory chain	Up regulation

9.2.6. LLLT- Anti Inflammatory Effects

There is substantial evidence that red and infrared LLLT demonstrates a dose-dependent anti-inflammatory effect. Inflammatory cytokines, namely, prostaglandin E2 (PGE2), tumour necrosis factor-alpha (TNF-α), cyclooxygenase 2 (COX-2), and interleukin 1 beta (IL-1β) can be repressed by exposure to LLLT [57].

Dose–response patterns for LLLT anti-inflammatory effects: Scrutiny of wavelengths between 632 nm and 904 nm has shown induction of considerable anti-inflammatory effects in biological tissues. The median value for laser mean optical output was 25 mW. Lower limits for anti-inflammatory effects were found to be 0.6 J/cm^2 in animal studies, and the lower limit for irradiation time was 16 seconds. Median irradiation time was 80 seconds in animal studies, but one study reported a significantly better effect when 3 J/cm^2 was delivered at low power density (5 mW/cm^2) over a longer period of time (600 seconds) than at high power density (50 mW/cm^2) over a shorter period of time (60 seconds). Two studies reported significantly better anti-inflammatory effects when doses were equal, but they were delivered with longer irradiation times. Upper limits for anti-inflammatory effects remain uncertain for power densities above 135 mW/cm^2 and doses above 15 J. Both infrared and red lasers were significantly better than LEDs emitting red wavelength in the same experimental model [58].

The effect can be compromised if LLLT is combined with glucocorticoid steroids, which have a negative interaction with LLLT. Red and infrared LLLT is administered with mean laser outputs ranging from 10 to 100 mW and irradiation times from 20 to 60 seconds, and doses between 0.6 and 9.6 J, reduce inflammation significantly and are as effective as NSAIDs in cell and animal studies [10].

When one laser output is known, LLLT doses can be easily calculated using the formula:

(Mean output mW *irradiation time sec)/1000= Dose (J) [11, 56].

Most of the literature has been performed with the laser probe in a fixed position during treatment. As a rule of thumb, each irradiated point will cover about 1–2 cm^3 of the pathology, so one should ensure that a sufficient number of points are selected to cover the entire pathology. If LLLT is used as recommended in WALT (World Association for Laser Therapy) guidelines, then it is an effective and safe therapy [10].

9.2.7. LLLT- Analgesia

In vivo studies of the analgesic effect of LLLT on nerves supplying the oral cavity have demonstrated that LLLT decreases the firing frequency of nociceptors, with a threshold effect seen in terms of the irradiance required to exert maximal suppression. *In vivo*, LLLT selectively inhibits a range of nociceptive signals arising from peripheral nerves, including neuronal discharges elicited by pinch, cold, heat stimulation, and chemical irritation [59]. In contrast, neuronal discharges induced by brush stimulation are not affected by LLLT. There is some evidence that laser irradiation may selectively target fibres conducting at slow velocities, particularly afferent axons from nociceptors. While the target tissues can be irradiated directly to elicit analgesic effects, an alternative approach is to irradiate target skin points used in acupuncture or acupressure. There have been claims that successful analgesia following oral surgery can be achieved with all major LLLT wavelengths from 632 nm to 904 nm [60, 61].

9.3. Principles of Photodynamic Therapy

Photodynamic therapy (PDT) is a comparatively novel treatment modality, incorporating the administration of a *photosensitizer* followed by local illumination with visible light of specific wavelength(s). In the *presence of oxygen*, the light illumination of photosensitizer can lead to a series of photochemical reactions and consequently the generation of *cytotoxic species*. The *nature, quantity, and location of PDT-induced cytotoxic species determine the nature and consequences of PDT treatment* [10-12].

9.3.1. Historical Background

The ability of visible light to destroy living organisms in the presence of a photosensitizer was initially observed by *Oscar Raab* more than 100 years ago while working on the effect of acridine on the behaviour of paramecia [62]. *Hermann von Tappeiner* et al. later recognized that oxygen was essential for the cytotoxic effect and he introduced the term *Photodynamic Therapy (Photodynamische Wirkung)* to describe this phenomenon [63, 64]. Modern photodynamic therapy (PDT) only began to form in the 1960s after *Richard Lipson and Edward Baldes* at Mayo Clinic (USA) reported that neoplastic tissues containing porphyrin mixtures could fluoresce under ultraviolet light irradiation [65].

9.3.2. Photosensitizers

A decisive element in PDT is the incorporation of a suitable photosensitizer. In general, photosensitizers can be divided into three broad families based on their origin and structure: [4]

1. *porphyrin-based photosensitizer* (e.g., Photofrin, ALA/PpIX, BPD-MA),
2. *chlorophyll-based photosensitizer* (e.g., chlorins, bacteriochlorins, purpurins), and
3. *dye* (e.g., phthalocyanine series, phenothiazinium series).
    - Traditionally, the porphyrins and those photosensitizers developed in the 1970s and early 1980s (e.g., Photofrin and

other haematoporphyrin derivatives) are called *first-generation photosensitizers*.

- Porphyrin derivatives or synthetics (e.g., ALA) made since the late 1980s are called *second-generation photosensitizers*.
- *Third-generation photosensitizers* generally refer to the modifications such as biologic conjugates (e.g., antibody conjugate, liposome conjugate) and built-in photo quenching or bleaching capability [66].

Clinically relevant criteria of an ideal photosensitizer include the following: [4]

1. A commercially available pure chemical.
2. Low dark toxicity but strong photocytotoxicity.
3. Good selectivity towards targeted cells.
4. Strong absorption of long-wavelength light.
5. Rapid removal from the body and therefore less skin photosensitization.
6. Ease of administration through various routes.

9.3.2.1. Light Applicators

The first light sources used in PDT were non-coherent light sources (e.g., conventional arc lamps). Non-coherent light sources are safer, easy to use, can be used in combination with optical filters, are less expensive, and produce a wide spectrum of wavelengths to accommodate different photosensitizers. The counted disadvantages include thermal effect, low light intensity, and difficulty in controlling light dose. Emerging Light-emitting diode (LED) can generate high-energy light of desired wavelengths and can be assembled in different geometries and sizes. The most widespread PDT light sources are lasers, which produce high energy monochromatic light with a narrow bandwidth [67, 68].

Four light delivery modes are commonly used in clinical settings: [4]

1. *Front superficial irradiation* - a uniform irradiance incident beam delivered to a surface by a microlens fiber externally.
2. *Cavity superficial irradiation* - an isotropic source centered in a spherical cavity and delivering light to the cavity surface.
3. *Cylindrical superficial irradiation* - a cylindrical diffuser source centered in a cylindrical lumen.
4. *Cylindrical interstitial irradiation* - a cylindrical diffuser source embedded in the target tissue.

9.3.3. Mechanisms of PDT Action

9.3.3.1. Photophysics and Photochemistry [69, 70, 71]

Upon capturing light energy, the photosensitizer can be excited to a triplet state *via* the intersystem crossing process. While returning to the ground state the excited photosensitizer can undergo Type I and Type II reactions. In a Type I reaction, the excited photosensitizer can interact directly with certain substrates, such as the cellular component or a molecule, and transfer a proton or an electron to form a radical anion or radical cation, respectively. These radicals may further interact with oxygen to produce oxygenated products. In a Type II reaction, the excited photosensitizer can transfer its energy directly to molecular oxygen to generate singlet oxygen. Singlet oxygen is highly destructive because it reacts with most organic molecules at almost diffusion-controlled rates, that is its rate of reaction is limited only by the speed at which it diffuses. It is involved in addition reactions to enes and dienes, forming hydroperoxides and endoperoxides, which can further propagate free radical chain reactions. Both reactions are oxygen-dependent and can occur simultaneously, and the ratio and yield of radicals are affected by photosensitizer properties and tissue partial oxygen pressure ($p0_2$). The generation of reactive oxygen species (ROS) can subsequently induce therapeutic effects, such as cell death (necrosis and apoptosis) and tissue destruction, through several well-known mechanisms. Also, photobleaching is light-mediated destruction of photosensitizer, and it is not clear whether photobleaching affects PDT activity.

9.3.3.2. Direct Cytotoxicity [4, 72, 73]

PDT-induced cytotoxic species have a short lifetime and only act within a limited distance. Therefore, the uptake and sub cellular localization of photosensitizer by tumor or other cells is critical in PDT-mediated direct cytotoxicities. The sub cellular localization is determined by the chemical properties, formulation, concentration, and delivery route of the photosensitizing drug, the microenvironment of the lesion, and to a certain degree the phenotype of the target cell. The plasma membrane, intracellular membranes, and organelles, such as the endoplasmic reticulum, Golgi apparatus, lysosomes, mitochondria and nucleus, have been identified as sub cellular PDT targets for many photosensitizers. Some photosensitizers distribute very broadly in these membranes and organelles while some distribute specifically in lysosomes or mitochondria. Some might redistribute during light irradiation. The cell genotype, photosensitizer sub cellular location, and the PDT dose might determine whether cell death occurs by apoptosis or necrosis. In general, the mode of cell death switches from apoptosis to necrosis with the increase of the intensity of the insult. High-dose PDT-induced apoptosis might be a stochastic rather than a threshold effect. Interestingly, some researchers show that sub threshold low-dose ALAPDT can induce selective apoptosis of the tumor cells, without detectable (apoptotic or necrotic) damage to the normal cells. This might offer the possibility of treating patients with low-dose ALA-PDT to minimize PDT damages to the normal tissue. Two major apoptotic pathways have been characterized: the death receptor-mediated, or extrinsic pathway, and the mitochondria-mediated apoptosis, or intrinsic pathway. In addition to the activation of the molecular mechanisms leading to direct cell death, PDT may also initiate some metabolic reactions that could protect cells from oxidative damage. Although such advances help the rational design and choice of photosensitizers, the golden standard of evaluation of the efficacy of clinical PDT still relies on the gross response of the lesion or disease to PDT. For instance, in tumor ablation, the typical clinically relevant response or biological endpoint would be acute tumor necrosis, the duration, and rate of this response, and the length of the tumor-free period. These might be affected by not only the direct cytotoxicity but also by other PDT effects as well as the tumor sensitivity to various PDT effects.

9.3.3.3. Vascular Effect

1. It has long been recognized since the early 1980s that an additional indirect mechanism, coexisting with the primary direct cytotoxicity of PDT, is the vascular effect in which vascular damage causes ischaemic death and therefore provides another approach to treat solid tumours [74].
2. Irradiation of photosensitizers, either confined in the blood circulation or accumulated in endothelial cells or bound to the vessel walls, results in collateral damage to endothelial cells. The PDT-induced direct damage to endothelial cells can be characterized by the loss of tight junctions between cells and exposure to vascular basement membranes. This primary damage within the vessel lumen leads to the formation of thrombogenic sites and initiation of a physiological cascade of reactions such as platelet aggregation, the release of vasoactive molecules, leukocyte adhesion, increase in vascular permeability, and vessel constriction. Microvascular collapse, blood flow stasis, and tissue haemorrhages can lead to severe persistent post-PDT tumour hypoxia and long-term tumour control [10].
3. Photosensitizers bound to carrier molecules, such as albumin, HDL, or LDL, appear to have an active affinity to endothelial cells and tumour microvascular endothelium because of the existence of specific receptors in high numbers in these structures. This might be an additive factor in photosensitizer uptake and retention in the tumour tissue [75].

4. Although one can expect that the localization of photosensitizer in both vascular and target cell compartments might produce a stronger combination effect, 33 several investigations have also shown that tumour response to vascular-targeted PDT does not correlate with the cellular concentration of photosensitizer in the treated tumour. Therefore, in vascular-targeted PDT mode, the light irradiation should be applied during photosensitizer infusion and continued after the completion of infusion so as to centre the light delivery period around the peak of the plasma concentration of photosensitizer and hence, putatively, should be maximizing the effect [75].

9.3.3.4. Immune Responses

1. PDT causes noticeable but short-term and reversible immune suppression under certain experimental conditions. However, unlike chemotherapy and irradiation therapy, PDT does not cause severe negative effects on the host immune system. Antitumor immune process and enhancement of host immune system might play important roles in secondary cytotoxicity, long-term tumour control, and/or complete tumour response to PDT, although these effects are not necessarily lethal to all tumour cells or relevant to the initial tumour ablation [76].
2. *In vivo,* animal studies show that pro-inflammatory damages formed in cellular membranes and the blood vessel walls of treated sites, start to recruit neutrophils, mast cells, and monocytes/macrophages after PDT. These cells can also release more inflammatory mediators to enable massive recruitment of immune cells to the tumour site. These immune cells and nonspecific immune effector cells have a profound impact on the PDT-mediated destruction of the tumour. PDT can also activate the expression and production of several cytokines, such as IL-lp, IL-2, IL-6, IL-10, TNF-a, and G-CSF. These cytokines play

important roles in regulating host immune responses involving both lymphoid and non-lymphoid cells [77].

3. Recent human trial suggests that PDT could enhance the uptake and presentation of tumor antigens by tumour-associated antigen-presenting cells (APC) and could ensure lymphocyte involvement. Complement-activating agents may further enhance the antitumor effect of PDT. PDT-treated tumour cell lysates can be effective tumour vaccines, although the mechanism for enhancement of host anti-tumour immune responses to PDT vaccines is still unclear. These advances in understanding PDT-induced immune responses might lead to an attempt to optimize PDT-mediated anti-tumour modality through the modulation of important inflammatory/immune mediators. While immune responses may be considered as a secondary effect of PDT, a combination modality designed to activate host immunological stimulation has been pursued. An effective approach is to use immunoadjuvants. This can in general enhance the host immune system and improve long-term tumour control in animal models [78, 79, 80].

9.4. Lasers in Recurrent Aphthous Ulcerations

The recurrent aphthous ulcer (RAU) is the most common ulcerative lesion found in the oral cavity. Afflicting the oral non-keratinized mucosa, they are painful, have a rounded appearance, gray/white in color, with an erythematous rim. The aetiology remains unknown; among patient factors are genetic predisposition, local trauma, medications, allergy, hormonal changes, stress, and immunological abnormalities. These tend to heal spontaneously in 10–15 days. They may be single or multiple, scattered in several areas; the pain can be intense enough to prevent feeding, speech, and oral hygiene [81].

Table 11. Use of Lasers in treatment of Recurrent Aphthous Ulcers

Authors	Type of Study	Laser Type	Laser Parameters	Results
Narjiss Akerzou et al. (2018) [84]	Case report	Diode laser 915 nm	2 W, CW, noncontact mode, 300s/cm^2	Complete remission over a period of 5 days
Rocca Jean-Paul et.al. (2018) [85]	Comparative study	1. ER:YAG 2. diode, 635 nm 3. diode, 808 nm 4. diode, 450 nm	PW, 60s, 76.43 J/cm^2 CW, 30s x3, 36 J/cm^2 CW, 60s, 50 J/cm^2 CW, 60s, 17 J/cm2	Er:YAG showed pain relief immediately after laser application, but the pain after 3 days of treatment was quite the same as before-treatment. With 808 nm and 450 nm improvement after application was observed, and gradually improved until 7 days after the treatment. Best results were obtained with 635 nm diode laser.
Hasan Guney Yilmaz et al. (2017) [81]	Randomized controlled split-mouth clinical study	Er,Cr:YSGG laser	Hard tissue mode, 0.25W, repetition rate 20 kHz, pulse duration of 140 μs, without water, 10% air at 5 J/cm^2, non-contact mode, 20 s per surface	A statistically significant difference between the scores of VAS and HRAS was found for all control days except day 10th according to the intergroup comparisons. Based on these findings, Er,Cr:YSGG laser application at 0.25W without water may be appropriate to reduce pain and accelerate the healing of RAS.
Fernando Alves Vale et al. (2015) [86]	Systematic review	GaAlAs laser, 809 nm	60mW,1800Hz, 80 s per treatment, 6.3 J/cm^2	Complete resolution of the ulcers in the active group required 3.05 ± 1.10 days, compared with 8.90 ± 0.45 days in the sham control group. Compared with the sham group, the authors found the complete healing time for the LLLT group to be highly significant.
Margit Albrektson et.al. (2014) [87]	Single-blinded placebo-controlled, randomized control trial	GaAlAs laser 809 nm	60 mW, 1800 Hz, 80s per treatment; 6.3 J/cm^2	VAS score decreased (day 0 until day 2) from 84.7 to 31.5 (LLLT) and from 81.7 to 76.1 (placebo) ($p < .0001$). LLLT relieved the difficulty of drinking, eating, and brushing teeth.

Table 11. (Continued)

Authors	Type of Study	Laser Type	Laser Parameters	Results
Nasrin Zand et al. (2012) [88]	Pilot study	non-thermal, non-ablative CO_2 laser therapy (NACLT)	1 W, defocused continuous mode, 5–10 s	The healing period was significantly shorter in ulcers treated by laser than in those treated with placebo ($p = 0.02$). There were no visible side effects after NACLT and during follow-up periods. Single NACLT could be used to promote wound healing in minor aphthous ulcers ($p = 0.02$).

RAU lesions follow a sequence of stages that can be described as: (1) prodromal – the presence of symptoms but without any visible clinical signs; (2) preulcerative – initial presentation usually with erythema and slight oedema; (3) ulcerative – formation of the epithelial defect; (4) healing – symptom abatement and progressive healing; and (5) remission – no evidence of lesions. Also, RAU has three clinical presentations: minor aphthous ulcers, major aphthous ulcers, and herpetiform ulcers [10, 11].

9.4.1. Laser Irradiation Protocol

The primary goals of therapy of RAU are relief of pain, reduction of ulcer duration, and restoration of normal oral function. The secondary goals include reduction in frequency and severity of recurrences and maintenance of remission [82, 83].

9.4.1.1. Pain Relief

As the lesion starts to heal, there are a few days (3–5 days) when the main symptom is severe pain. At this time, the patient seeks pain relief. LLLT is the only therapy capable of promoting immediate analgesia with no side effects, being a great clinical differential for dentists and improving the patient's perception. Also, when LLLT is performed at this time, the duration of the RAU cycle will also be reduced. The LLLT protocol is daily infrared laser irradiation (2.0–3.0 J per point) until remission of symptoms [10].

9.4.1.2. Acceleration of Wound Healing

The LLLT protocol is daily red laser irradiation (0.5–1.0 J per point) until complete lesion healing.

9.4.1.3. RAU Prevention

LLLT can be also used when the patient has no RAU manifestations. LLLT stimulates the immune system and increases the resistance of the mucosa to ulcer formation. The LLLT protocol is weekly infrared or red laser irradiation (2.0–3.0 J per point) for 10 weeks in all regions of high incidence of RAU manifestations (the patient should be asked to indicate the more critical areas). The following are useful tips for LLLT: [10]

1. An anti-inflammatory and analgesic effect dose should be used on and around the lesion;
2. The number of points of irradiation can be increased until the patient reports pain relief of at least 90% (the patient should be asked to rate their perception of pain from 0% to 100% before and after irradiation);
3. As radiation scatters around the lesion while performing the analgesic protocol, this lower scattered energy will also improve the healing process.
4. Whenever possible, laser irradiation must be perpendicular to avoid loss of energy.

A comparative collation of recent studies demonstrating the use of lasers in the treatment of recurrent aphthous ulcerations has been summarized in Table 11.

9.5. Lasers in Burning Mouth Syndrome

The Burning mouth syndrome (BMS) has been classified as a distinct disease in 2004 by the International Headache Society, which defined the primary form as "a feeling of intraoral burning sensation for which no medical or dental cause can be found" [90]. The diagnosis is mainly by exclusion. Usually, the distribution of oral burning is bilateral, although it does not follow anatomical structures. The most commonly affected site is the tongue, especially in the anterior region, followed by the lips, hard palate, mucosa, and oropharynx. A variety of psychosocial features and personality disorders are seen in BMS patients, such as alexithymic traits, cancerophobia, somatization, obsession–compulsion, personal sensitivity, hostility, psychoticism, and social isolation, as well as significantly higher adverse early life experiences and a higher mean score for anxiety and depression, compared with appropriate controls. However, as with other chronic pain syndromes, these findings do not distinguish between cause and effect. BMS appears to be more prevalent in middle-aged and older women (mean age, 50–60 years), with a female-to male ratio varying from 3:1 to 16:1. Its pathogenic mechanisms and aetiological factors are largely unknown. Some researchers have suggested that the disorder may be a manifestation of somatization, while others have reported it to be more closely related to neuropathic pain than to somatoform chronic pain syndromes [11, 90, 91].

9.5.1. Laser Irradiation Protocol

BMS patients should be subjected to a weekly session of LLLT for 10 weeks, totalling ten sessions. The laser irradiation used has a continuous wavelength of 660 nm, power of 40 mW, energy of 20 J/cm2, with 0.4 J per point. Before irradiation, the affected area must be cleaned and dried with gauze. Each point of irradiation must be precise, with approximately 1 cm between each point, and irradiation duration of 10 seconds for each. For each affected anatomical area, depending on its size, three to six irradiation points should be used. The burning intensity should be relieved in all sessions according to the visual analogue scale (VAS). The assessment of this intensity should be performed immediately before and immediately after laser irradiation in each LLLT session. A comparison between these two assessments will yield the effect of LLLT [10, 11].

9.5.1.1. LLLT in BMS [4, 10]

1. Due to its differential properties, such as monochromaticity, coherence, and directivity, the laser can deposit a large quantity of energy in biological tissues with extreme precision.

Table 12. Use of lasers in Burning Mouth Syndrome

Authors	Type of Study	Type of Laser	Laser Parameters	Results
Juliana-Cassol Spanemberg et al. (2019) [90]	Double-blind, randomized, controlled clinical trial	GaAlAs 808 nm ± 5 nm (infrared)	200 mW , 1.97W/cm^2 , 3 J per point and application time 15 seconds per point For 2-week sessions of LLLT for 4 weeks	The study obtained levels of significance for the improvement variable for the laser group at two-month follow-up ($p = 0.0038$); marginally significant in dry mouth, dysgeusia, pain, and the treatment ($p = .053$); no statistically significant differences between the groups before or after the treatment for psychological profiles.
Miroslav Sikora et al. (2018) [91]	Pilot study	GaAlAs 830 nm	100 mW, chopped mode (switched on: 800 ms, switched off : 1 ms), 12 J/cm^2, non-contact mode; repeated every day except for weekend for 14 days (10sessions). Every session lasted for 5 minutes.	Significant decrease in pain symptoms (VAS) in both LLLT switched on and LLLT switched off groups ($p < 0.05$). Neither LLLT switched off or switched on improved the oral health impact on the quality of life scale OHIP-CRO 14 scores.
Sadeq Ali Al-Maweri et al. (2016) [92]	Systematic Review	Diode laser 630- 980 nm	20-300 mW, 10 seconds-15 minutes	The majority of the studies showed that laser therapy seemed to be effective in reducing pain in BMS patients.
Norberto Nobuo Sugaya et al. (2015) [93]	A randomized, placebo-controlled study	AsGaAI 790 nm	20 mW , 6 J/cm^2	The results were categorized according to the percentage of symptom level variation and showed a statistically better response in the Laser group only in two categories (excellent E and no burning NB) of the control checkpoints ($p = 0.02$).
Lucia de Fatima C. dos Santos et al. (2014) [94]	Prospective study	660 nm	40 mW, 10 J cm^2 and 0.4 J per point, 10 s for 10 weeks	All volunteers reported reduced burning intensity in all sessions when compared to the previous one and a reduction in VAS scores by up to 49% in the last clinical session when compared to the first session.

Authors	Type of Study	Type of Laser	Laser Parameters	Results
Sonja Pezelj-Ribarić et al. (2013) [90]	Case-control study	5 days in a week for four consecutive weeks with 685-nm gallium–aluminium–arsenic diode laser	30 mW, 3.0 J/cm^2, for 10 min, CW	In the experimental group, levels of TNF-α measured before LLLT were significantly greater than TNF-α levels following therapy ($p < 0.001$). Levels of IL-6 before LLLT were also significantly greater than after LLLT ($p < 0.001$). In the control group, no significant difference was found in the levels of TNF-α and IL-6 before and after the application of LLLT.

2. LLLT promotes cellular biomodulation in healing injuries (proliferation of fibroblasts, collagen synthesis, and the regeneration of bone and nerve tissues). Laser irradiation promotes immediate relief in areas affected by burning through the formation of a greater quantity of β-endorphin by the glial cells and a decrease in the production of prostaglandins. The action of the laser beam on the cyclooxygenases regulates the transformation of arachidonic acid, as well as provides a biostimulatory effect by increasing mitochondrial ATP and thus optimizing the speed of regeneration in the affected area.

A comparative collation of recent studies demonstrating the use of lasers in the treatment of burning mouth syndrome has been summarized in Table 12.

9.6. Lasers in Temporomandibular Disorders

Temporomandibular dysfunction (TMD) is a group of disorders that affect the masticatory muscles, temporomandibular joint (TMD), and associated structures. It is the most prevalent clinical entity involving the masticatory apparatus and is the main cause of pain of non-dental origin in the facial region. When there is an imbalance in this dynamic system, a wide range of clinical problems arises; musculoskeletal disorders develop very characteristic signs and symptoms, the main one being muscle and/or joint pain, which implies the limitation of mandibular movements. In addition to these, other symptoms may or may not develop concomitantly, such as cephalea, cervical pain, joint noise, muscle fatigue, dizziness, hearing loss, and tinnitus [101]. The treatment of these disorders is multidisciplinary and is aimed at the control of pain symptoms through drug therapy, at treating the functional limitation through physiotherapy treatment of the masticatory muscles, stress control, using cognitive behavioural therapy, massage and relaxation techniques, occlusal plaques up to complex surgical and prosthetic rehabilitation [95, 96].

9.6.1. Mechanism of Action [4, 10, 11]

1. Epicentres of pain: On the basis of Arthroscopic studies, the concept that capsular, synovial, and retrodiscal tissue inflammation is the basis of the pain in the joint region in TMD. Also in pain of myogenous origin due to increased muscle activity, the circulatory system does not support the drainage of metabolites and oxygen supply to the hypoxic areas, leading to a local accumulation of toxins and subsequent inflammatory response.
2. If the correct parameters are used, LLLT can provide analgesic and anti-inflammatory effects by:
   - stimulation of endogenous opiate release
   - decrease of the neuronal cell membrane permeability
   - decrease in the release of pain agents at pathological sites
   - increase in ATP production
   - increase in local oxygenation.
3. Pain reduction attributed to a drop in the level of prostaglandin E2: Studies using varying doses of energy and power output have shown a reduction in PGE2 after LLLT in ligament cell cultures and the articulation of animals. Probably, the reason can be attributed to the inhibition of the enzyme that synthesizes PGE2, the cyclooxygenase-2.
4. The action of LLLT on neuronal cells: selective inhibition of nociceptive signals and regulation of the microcirculation causes analgesia. A reduction in oedema and an increase in cellular metabolism have also been reported. LLLT has a systemic effect that may decrease the perception of pain by altering the sensorial input to a patient's central nervous system [26] When applied to cases of muscle pain in TMD, studies have described its

analgesic effect: it increases the level of beta-endorphins, decreases the release of histamine and bradykinin, increases lymphatic flow, decreases oedema and pain substance release, increases blood supply, decreases the duration of inflammation, and consequently relaxes muscles.

9.6.1.1. Laser Irradiation Protocol

Table 13. Treatment protocol for articular symptoms [10]

Active medium	Diode laser (AsGaAl)
Wavelength	808 nm (infrared)
Power output	100 mW
Spot size	0.028 cm^2
Irradiance	3.5 W/cm^2
Energy per point	2.8 J
Energy density	100 J/cm^2
Time	28 s
Number of points	4
Frequency	Continuous
Mode	In contact
Number of sessions	12 (three a week)

Table 14. Treatment protocol for muscular symptoms [10]

Active medium	Diode laser (AsGaAl)
Wavelength	808 nm (infrared)
Power output	100 mW
Spot size	0.028 cm^2
Irradiance	3.5 W/cm^2
Energy per point	2.8 J
Energy density	100 J/cm^2
Time	28 s
Number of points	1 per 1.5 cm^2 of the muscle in pain
Frequency	Continuous
Mode	In contact
Number of sessions	12 (three a week)

The LLLT parameters for TMD treatment should be determined according to the level of commitment of the articular or muscular structures, clinical signs and symptoms, time of evolution of the disease, and individual physical aspects (Table 13, 14).

9.6.1.2. Considerations for LLLT of TMJ [10]

1. The LLLT should be applied around the articular capsule with consideration for the presence of numerous nociceptors in the periauricular tissue (disc, capsular ligaments, and retrodiscal tissue).
2. TMJ internal derangements are often associated with pain due to the inflammatory process stretching or disrupting the TMJ collateral ligaments. The most common areas affected by muscle pain in TMD are the masseter and anterior temporal muscles.
3. The precise points of applications should be determined according to the complaint and the anatomy of each patient (Figure 11).
4. The LLLT can be applied to the muscle that the patient indicates to be painful upon compression, or trigger points or acupuncture points.
5. Usually, irradiation is applied between the origin, body, or insertion of the masseter muscle (up to three irradiation points) and the anterior, middle, and posterior temporal muscle (up to two points each) (Figure 12, 13).
6. Based on the scattering pattern of infrared low-power lasers, the application points should be 1.5 cm^2 apart to avoid energy overlap.
7. The World Association for Laser Therapy recommends two to three sessions of LLLT per week, over 3–5 weeks. It is also important that the treatment is sequential, so the cumulative effect of LLLT can be achieved.

A comparative collation of recent studies demonstrating the use of lasers in the treatment of Temporomandibular disorders has been summarized in Table 15.

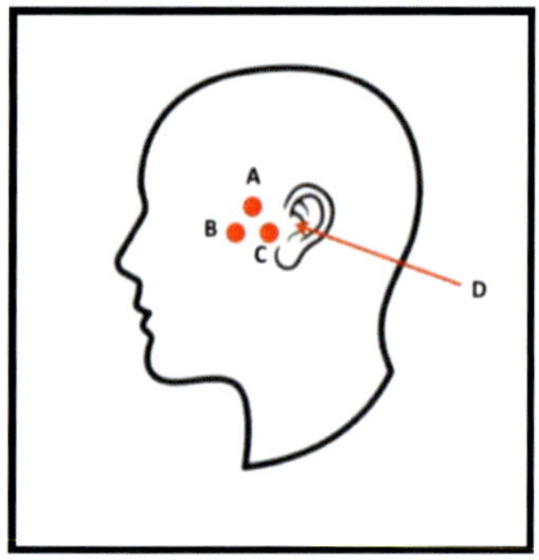

Figure 11. Points of laser application for the TMJ: (A) above the condyloid process, (B) anterior to the condyloid process, (C) posterior to the condyloid process, and (D) an intra-auricular point towards the joint.

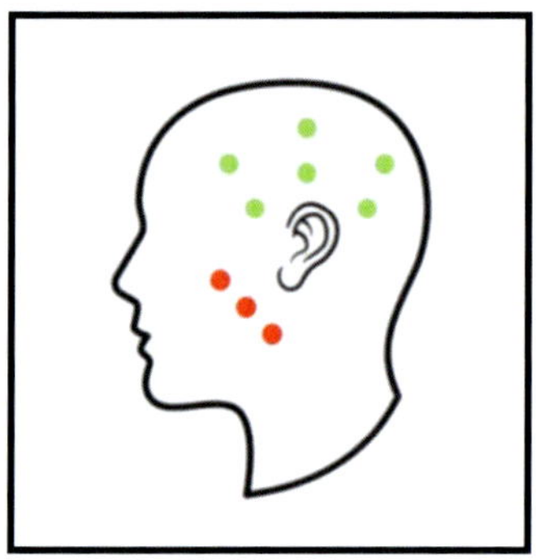

Figure 12. Possible points of laser application for the masseter and temporalis muscles.

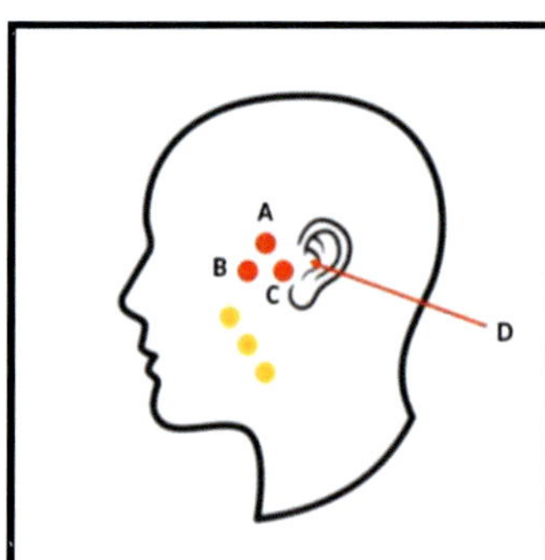

Figure 13. Possible points of laser application for the masseter muscle and TMJ.

Table 15. Use of lasers in Temporomandibular Disorders

Authors	Type of Study	Laser Type	Laser Parameters	Results
Fernanda Thomé Brochado et al. (2018) [97]	Randomized clinical trial	GaAlAs diode laser 808 nm	100 mW, 13.3 J/cm^2, and 4 J per point, 3.33 W/cm^2	Seven evaluations were performed with VAS, RDC/TMD Axis I and II, and BAI. Treatment did not promote modification in the intensity of chronic pain. Manual Therapy promoted improvement in 5 functions, PBM in 2, and CT in 1 ($p < 0.001$). BAI revealed a reduction in anxiety ($p \leq 0.05$). All were able to promote pain relief, improve mandibular function, and reduce the negative psychosocial aspects and levels of anxiety in TMD patients. The combination of PBM and MT did not promote an increase in the effectiveness of both therapies alone.
Gang-Zhu Xu et al. (2018) [98]	Systematic Review with Meta-Analysis	GaAlAs GaAs Nd:YAG InGaAlP Diode	Shortest wavelength -632.8 nm and the longest was 1064 nm. Laser dosage varied from 1.5 J/cm2 to 112.5 J/cm^2; four studies did not report the dosage	Positive effects of LLLT on pain relief, VAS score, or the change of VAS score between the baseline and final follow-up; discrepant about effects of high or low doses. TMJ function outcomes - overall effect favored LLLT over placebo.
Rosana Mengue Maggi Borges et al. (2018) [99]	Randomized, double-blind, placebo-controlled clinical trial	AlGaAs laser 830 nm	CW, 8 J/cm^2 , 60 J/cm^2 , 105 J/cm^2; 30mW/cm^2, 3× week/10 sessions	Mouth opening increased in the 8-J/cm^2 group from 10.49 ± 4.68 to 15.40 ± 6.43 degrees, and in the right protrusion from 9.80 ± 4.2 to 12.56 ± 5.40 ($p < 0.05$). All groups significantly decreased pain ($p < 0.05$). 830-nm laser photobiomodulation was effective in reducing TMD pain and symptoms at all doses tested. Only the doses of 8 J/cm^2 were effective regarding maximal opening and protrusion of the mandible.

Table 15. (Continued)

Authors	Type of Study	Laser Type	Laser Parameters	Results
Nermin Demirkol et al. (2018) [100]	Comparative study	Nd:YAG (1064 nm) Diode laser (810 nm)	Nd:YAG: 0.25W, 8 J/cm^2 , 20s Diode laser: 8 J/cm^2, 0.25W, 9s five times per week, for a total of 10 sessions	There were statistically significant differences in VAS scores in Nd:YAG ($p = 0.001$) and 810 nm diode laser groups ($p = 0.005$), but no difference in the placebo group ($p = 0.065$). Both the Nd:YAG and 810 nm diode lasers were effective for the treatment of subjective tinnitus related to TMDs.
Marcos Fernando Xisto Braga Cavalcanti et al. (2016) [101]	Comparative study	GaAlAs infrared laser diode 780 nm	35.0 J/cm^2, for 20 sec, thrice a week, for 4 weeks	Compared to physiotherapeutic and drug protocol, LLL treatment is effective to control pain associated with TMD.
Simel Ayyildiz et al. (2015) [102]	Case report	Diode laser 685 nm	6.2 J/cm2, 30s, 3 times a week for 1 month	Both cases reported a gradual increase in maximum mouth opening, right and left excursions post-treatment. The first case had a little relapse 6 months later.
Nabeel Sayed et al. (2013) [103]	Longitudinal interventional study	Gallium arsenide semi conductive diode laser 904 nm	0.6 W, 60 s, 4 J/cm2; 3 times a week for 2 weeks for 6 months	Pain intensity, number of tender points, joint sounds, and active range of motion showed positive improvement.

9.7. Lasers in Lymphatic Drainage of Oedema

LLLT has been shown to be capable of reducing inflammation in a wide variety of clinical situations, whether reducing the development of the oedema and migration of inflammatory cells or modulating the formation of inflammation-mediating substances. LLLT modifies some fundamental processes of aneurysm of the aorta, progressively increasing the cell proliferation of the smooth muscle and of the protein matrix, as well as the secretion of the matrix metalloproteinase. LLLT inhibits the generic expression of pro-inflammatory cytokines and interleukin-1β from irradiated cells. On the other hand, it has been suggested that LLLT promotes the early activation of the inflammatory phase of the tissue repair process, causing an exacerbation of signs and symptoms [104].

The inflammatory oedema results initially from the action of histamine, followed by the effect of kinins, and is potentiated by the action of prostaglandins (after approximately 5–6 hours). Throughout the first 24 hours, the prostaglandins are largely responsible for the extent of oedema. As with pain, the action of anti-inflammatory drugs is dependent on the reduction of the local production of prostaglandins. Prostaglandins are also important in the repair process. The efficacy of LLLT lies in the fact that it modulates the local production of such prostaglandins, and does not inhibit their production [10].

9.7.1. Laser Irradiation Parameters

The aim of LLLT is to activate the lymphatic drainage of a region where inflammation is established. Digital palpation of the lymph node chains will detect any altered surface lymph nodes where irradiation should be applied [4, 10, 11]

1. A laser that emits in the proximal infrared (preferably between 808 and 830 nm) region is indicated.

2. The tip of the equipment must be placed on the lymph nodes responsible for draining the affected region, as perpendicular to them as possible.
3. An energy dose of approximately 2 J, giving a fluency of approximately 70 J/cm^2, is given at each application point.
4. The number of sessions will depend on the duration of the inflammation (generally two to six sessions, with an interval of 2 days between sessions protocol is used).
5. The placement of the laser must always avoid the irradiation of critical regions, such as the thyroid gland. Therefore, when positioning the laser to irradiate the sub mental lymph nodes, care must be taken to direct the laser beam upwards, towards the sublingual region, and never downwards towards the thyroid gland.

A comparative collation of recent studies demonstrating the use of lasers in the treatment of lymphatic drainage of oedema has been summarized in Table 16.

9.8. Lasers in Herpes Infections

Herpes is one of the most common communicable diseases worldwide. It is colloquially called a cold sore or fever blister [108]. Apart from recurrent and painful disruptions, herpes infection is usually associated with massive psychosocial distress, shame, and uncomfortable feelings, due to a marred aesthetic appearance. HSV enters the host through the skin and mucosal surfaces, commonly the oral cavity, genital tract, and cornea of the eye, by means of direct contact with infected secretions [109]. The majority of primary infections are subclinical. The primary HSV-1 lesions appear as vesicles on the oral mucosa, often associated with pain and fever. After healing of lesions, in around 1–2 weeks, the virus is transported to the trigeminal ganglion and there remains latent until reactivation. The reactivation occurs when there is a decrease in the resistance of the immune system, such as an illness, prolonged exposure to sunlight, or cold weather, and most commonly, extended or acute periods of stress. In most cases (around 80%), the recurrent infections cause only salivary asymptomatic infection, but some patients develop a symptomatic process, where vesicles appear on the mucosa and/or skin of the face, usually associated with pain and itchiness. The vesicles rupture and coalesce after some days, forming crusts that can take 2 weeks to heal, depending on the lesion extension, and then the virus returns to latency [110]

Depending on the stage of the lesion, various modalities of phototherapy like Low Power Laser (LPL) therapy and Photodynamic Therapy (PDT) have been implemented with favourable results.

These have been summarized in Table 17.

9.9. Other Applications of LLLT

There have been many claims for the therapeutic effects of LLLT on a broad range of disorders, including the following:

1. Alveolar osteitis
2. Neurosensory recovery after injury to Inferior Alveolar Nerve
3. Bells palsy
4. Trigeminal neuralgia
5. Post-herpetic neuralgia
6. Oral lesions in Pemphigus
7. Oral lesions in Steven-Johnson's syndrome and Toxic Epidermal Necrolysis
8. Oral mucositis
9. Bisphosphonate induced Osteoradionecrosis
10. Pericoronitis

Table 16. Use of lasers for Lymphatic Drainage of Edema

Authors	Type of Study	Laser Type	Laser Parameters	Results
Leandro Lauriti et al. (2017) [105]	Pilot Study	Ga-Al-As 660 nm	108mW, 21.6 J/cm^2, 38197 mW/cm^2; exposure time, 200 sec per point, 10 points bilaterally. Photobiomodulation was performed in 15 sessions.	Improvements in the laser group in comparison with the sham group with regard to mandibular dynamics, a reduction in postoperative facial swelling, a reduction in pain, and an increase in bite force.
Abdelrahman E.M. Ezzat et al. (2016) [106]	Randomized double blinded clinical study	Diode laser 970 ± 15 nm	Continuous non-contact, 35 J/cm^2; local application of laser immediately after surgery. The treatment sessions were 3 with 30 s relaxation time between each consecutive session with a total time of 3 min	Preliminary results showed that low-level laser therapy is effective in the reduction of postoperative pain and oedema, and minimizing the need of analgesic medication after secondary palatal operations.
Cennet Neslihan Eroglu et al. (2016) [107]		Diode laser 940 nm	4 J/cm2, 0.5 watt/cm^2, contact mode, single session	A single-session LLLT that would be applied with a diode laser immediately after impacted tooth extraction might help patients to be less affected by postoperative trismus and swelling.

Table 17. Use of lasers for Herpes Infections

Authors	Phase	Method	Laser Type	Laser Parameters
Marotti et al. [111]	Vesicle	PDT	660–670 nm (red light)	MB 0.01% 5 min + 100 J/cm^2, 100 mW, 28 s/point, 2.8 J
Marotti et al. [112]	Crust	LPL	660–670 nm (red light)	20 J/cm^2, 40 mW, 14 s/point, 0.5 J/point, 4 sessions in 1 week
Bello-Silva et al. [113]	Crust	LPL	660–670 nm (red light)	3.8 J/cm^2, 10 mW, 10 s/point, daily during 10 days
de Paulo Eduardo et al. [114]	Crust	LPL	660–670 nm (red light)	4 J/cm^2, 50 mW
de Carvalho et al. [115]	Prodrome/latent	LPL	780–808 nm (infrared light)	4.5 J/cm^2, 60 mW, 3 s/point, 1 session/week for 10 weeks

9.9.1. LLLT in Alveolar Osteitis

Alveolar osteitis or Dry socket is a postoperative complication after tooth extraction, which often impedes the healing process. It occurs in 0.5 to 5% of normal extractions and 1 to 37.5% of mandibular third molar extractions. Various terminologies like alveolar osteitis, alveolitissicca dolorosa, septic sockets, and necrotic socket have been proposed. LLLT showed a significant increase in wound healing when compared to Alveogyl group. Both Low power red laser(LPRL) 660mm and Low power infrared laser (LPIRC) 810 mm showed a significant reduction in pain compared to subjects using Alveogyl. The 660 mm laser was most effective on the second and third days and hence low-level laser should be investigated as an alternative for the treatment of alveolar osteitis [117].

9.9.2. LLLT in Neurosensory Recovery after Injury to Inferior Alveolar Nerve

There have been many claims for the therapeutic effects of LLL treatment such as acceleration of wound healing, pain attenuation, restoration of normal neural function following injury, enhanced remodeling, and repair of bone, normalization of abnormal hormonal function, stimulation of endorphin release, and modulation of the immune system. Tuncer Ozen et al. [118] used gallium-aluminium-arsenide (GaAlAs) LLL in patients with neurosensory impairment, and they reported both subjective and objective improvement in IAN after LLL treatment. Clinical neurosensory tests (the brush stroke directional discrimination test, 2-point discrimination test) and a subjective assessment of neurosensory function using a visual analogue scale) were used before and after treatment, and the responses were plotted over time, showing favourable results.

9.9.3. LLLT in Bells Palsy

For LLLT, a gallium–arsenide diode (GaAs) laser (BTL-5000 laser) can be used with infrared probes of 830 nm wavelength and 100 mW output power, an average energy density of 10 J/cm^2, frequency of 1 KHz, and a duty cycle of 80%. The laser can be placed in direct contact with the superficial roots of the facial nerve on the affected side and was applied for 2 min and 5 s per point for 8 points with a total energy of 80 J. LLLT applied for a total of 18 treatment sessions over a period of 6 consecutive weeks (three sessions/week) has given encouraging results [119].

9.9.4. LLLT in Trigeminal Neuralgia

Vernon and Hasbun [120] reported a 61-year-old female with TN. They treated her with GaAlAs diode-laser (808 nm, 200 mW) with a protocol of every day irradiation with two days interval after each five days. A total of 20 sessions of exposure were performed. The patient reported no pain at the 12th session. In another study, Walker et al. [121] exposed the patients with a history of TN with He-Ne laser (1 mW, 632.5 nm, 20 Hz) in a double-blind study. The duration of exposure for each site was 20 seconds for skin overlying peripheral nerves and painful facial areas. The control group received no irradiation with a laser apparatus identical to the laser group. Both groups received irradiation three times a week for ten weeks. Laser therapy was associated with a significant reduction in the intensity and frequency of pain. Clinical studies of the effects of LLLT on injured nerves have revealed an increase in nerve function and improved capacity for myelin production. LLLT has also been shown to be effective for promoting axonal growth in injured nerves in animal models [11].

9.9.5. LLLT in Post-Herpetic Neuralgia

In one study, 18 outpatients suffering severe post-herpetic neuralgia (PHN) were exposed to low-power helium-neon (He-Ne) laser [122]. The investigators used four-grade estimation, visual analogue scale (VAS), and modified McGill pain questionnaire (m-MPQ) after every 10 of 50 irradiations to determine the efficacy of the treatment. Results showed that repeated irradiation with a low-power He-Ne laser is an effective and safe therapy for post-herpetic neuralgia. Mann et al. [123] investigated the efficacy of combi laser in 50 patients with PHN. In each patient, the laser therapy was given for 15 days with a period of 5 minutes and 6 seconds exposure for each appointment. The therapeutic effect of the laser was evaluated after the 5th, 10th and 15th days with a visual analogue scale (VAS). Patients started responding after the third day and after completion of therapy, 43 out of 50 showed great relief (76-100%), four cases showed good relief (51-75%), two cases with fair relief (26-50%), and one case with poor relief (1-25%). Moore et al. [124] performed a double-blind cross-over trial of low-level laser therapy (LLLT) in treatment of established PHN of at least 6 months duration with no response to conventional methods of treatment. Patients were treated with a gallium aluminium arsenide (GaAlAs) diode laser (830 nm: 60mW). Results demonstrated a significant reduction in the intensity and distribution of pain (74% of patients) due to a course of LLLT (4 consecutive laser treatments).

9.9.6. Oral Lesions in Pemphigus

Nasrin Zand et al. [125] used the CO_2 laser (10 600 nm; Lancet-2, Russia) operated at 1 W power, in a continuous defocused mode, 5-6 mm distant from the surface of the gel while scanning rapidly over the lesion with a circular motion. In each pass, the laser energy was delivered to a circle area of the lesion (nearly 1 cm diameter) for 5 seconds and repeated immediately if the contact pain of the lesion persisted. The gel was gently wiped between the passes, and a new layer of gel was placed on the lesion to prevent decrease of water content of the gel and tissue damage. The procedure was pain-free and no kind of anaesthesia was needed. The results of the trial proposed that a single session of NTCLT could immediately and significantly relieve pain in oral lesions of PV, without any visible thermal complications [125].

9.9.7. Oral Lesions in Steven-Jhonson's Syndrome and TEN

In a case reported by Alyne Simoes et al. [126], a 7-year-old male patient, diagnosed with SJ syndrome, underwent both extra- and intraoral Laser phototherapy. The extraoral therapy was delivered with a 660-nm InGaAlP laser (Twin Laser; MMOptics Ltd., SP, Brazil). The irradiation was delivered with the laser tip in direct contact with and perpendicular to the patient's oral mucosa and lips, and lesions on the patient's perioral skin were treated in the same way. The laser settings were 15mW and 3.8 J/cm^2, at energy of 0.15 J per treatment point and a laser-beam spot size of 0.04 cm^2 for 10 s per treatment point. The irradiance was 0.375W/cm^2. For intraoral LPT (Photon Laser DMC, Paulo, Brazil), because of the patient's difficulty in opening his mouth, a smaller spot size, 0.028 cm^2 per treatment point, was used for his oral lesions, at 100 mW and 7.1 J/cm^2, and with an irradiation time of 2 s per treatment point. The irradiance was 3.571W/cm^2. Lesions on the patient's tongue were treated with direct application of the laser tip, and areas of ulceration on the patient's oral mucosa were treated with the laser in the defocused mode. At 5 days after the initial session of LPT, the patient was able to eat gelatin, and on the following day, the number and severity of his intraoral lesions and his labial crusting and swelling had diminished. By 6 days after his initial session of LPT, most of the patient's intraoral lesions had disappeared, and the few that remained were painless; the patient was able to eat solid food by himself and was removed from the ICU. Ten sessions of LPT were conducted in the hospital. The patient underwent three further and consecutive sessions at the School of Dentistry, when complete healing of his oral lesions was observed. The outcome, in this case, suggests that LPT may be a new adjuvant modality for SJS complications. In a case reported by Amanda Leal Rocha et al. [127], LLLT was performed for a 9-year-old girl diagnosed with TEN. Intraoral and labial mucosa was irradiated with 9 per point energy with a red light 660 - nm, power of 100 mw. The laser settings were 66.66-133.33 J/cm^2 with a laser beam spot size of 0.03 cm^2 for 20-40 s/cm^2. The treatment was delivered daily with the laser tip in direct contact with and perpendicular to the affected area of the oral mucosa. The total irradiation time by session was 8 - 10 minutes depending on the affected area. They demonstrated that LLLT might be an effective treatment of TEN-related oral lesions. The therapy was well tolerated and might be considered as a routine protocol in the treatment of mucosal drug-induced reactions.

9.9.8. Oral Mucositis

Oral mucositis is one of the cytotoxic effects of anticancer therapies; the incidence is variable (30–100%) in relation to drugs and/or treatments used. Clinically it presents various aspects ranging from moderate redness of the mucosa and mild symptoms to serious cases with extensive ulcerations that cause functional limitations. The most severe manifestations cause the inability to perform vital functions such as feeding. The use of LLLT in both the treatment and the prevention of oral mucositis is well documented in scientific literature; Multinational Association of Supportive Care in Cancer (MASCC) [128] guidelines recommend laser therapy in the prevention of oral mucositis in patients receiving pre-transplant conditioning; suggested parameters are 660 nm wavelength, 40 mW power, and fluence 2 J/cm^2 (level II evidence), while guidelines cannot be drawn up for other populations and other wavelengths because of insufficient scientific evidence. Caution is required in the treatment of mucositis when it is due to the treatment of head and neck cancers, as the mechanism of action of LLLT on tissue differentiation/ proliferation and on cancer cells is not yet clear, and thus, the possibility of local invasion or metastasis or the possibility of having effects at a distance must be kept in mind. While the in vitro results show an increase in the proliferation of cancer cells, in vivo this has not been observed, maybe because of the *in vivo* potential anticancer immunological reactivity. Wavelengths of between 633 and 685 nm and between 780 and 830 nm are indicated as effective, with output from 10 to 150 mW, fluence from 2 to 6 J/ cm^2 (2 J/cm^2 for prevention, 4 J/cm^2 for the treatment), 2–3 applications per week. If mucositis is severe, applications are recommended daily until symptoms subside, if pulsed, output frequency < 100 Hz, intra- and extra-oral applications [129]. It is recommended to start treatment before mucositis onset, to intercept with laser therapy the various stages of the disease, and to continue until the end of the cycles of chemotherapy and radiotherapy; all the oral mucosa has to undergo photobiomodulation, extending when possible until the beginning of the pharynx [130].

9.9.9. Bisphosphonate Induced Osteoradionecrosis

The action of LLLT on bone, studied both in vitro and in vivo, is performed through the proliferation and differentiation of osteoblasts with increased calcium salt deposit which accelerate calcification, through the activation of MCM genes (mini-chromosome maintenance proteins) regulated by DNA replication and through type I collagen formation. The most commonly used wavelengths are in the range between 650 and 1064 nm, power density between 5 and 150 mW/cm^2, 30–60 s per point, and fluence between 0.3 and 9 J/cm^2. For 1064 nm wavelength, the parameters used are power 1.25 W, frequency 15 Hz, fibre 320 μ, PD 1562.5 W/cm^2, and fluence 7 J/cm^2. On average, laser sessions are 2/3 times per week [131].

9.9.10. Pericoronitis

Adding LLLT to the traditional treatment modalities results in a faster reduction of oedema and pain. A large area is involved and should be covered, not loally only. If fever and swelling below the mandible are involved, LLLT should not be applied until antibiotics have been used; the laser irradiation will improve local microcirculation, possibly spreading the infection into lower areas [12].

Chapter 10

LASERS IN ORAL POTENTIALLY MALIGNANT DISORDERS

10.1. INTRODUCTION TO LASERS IN ORAL POTENTIALLY MALIGNANT DISORDERS

The terminology for oral lesions that may have the potential to progress to malignancy has varied over the years. The term *premalignant* is commonly used and is widely understood, but it implies that an individual lesion may inevitably become malignant. However, the risk is only statistically increased, and therefore the term potentially malignant, which suggests that the progression to malignancy is only a potential risk, has become more widely accepted. *Potentially premalignant* is an alternative term that is in keeping with the concept that not all lesions—for example, leukoplakia—will have any potential to progress to malignancy and that the clinician is faced with a mucosal change that is only a potentially premalignant lesion. At a World Health Organization (WHO) workshop in 2007, it was also recommended that the distinction between potentially malignant lesions and conditions be abandoned in favor of a common term, *oral potentially malignant disorders (OPMDs)* and this has now been accepted in the latest WHO classification [132]. Traditional treatment has involved surgical excision with a scalpel, which has many disadvantages compared with laser excision or ablation procedures. The advantages of using a laser include better control of bleeding, less surgical time, more precise tissue removal, less morbidity and complications, and excellent healing with virtually no scarring. Many surgeons also believe that the cauterization effect of the laser on blood vessels and lymphatic channels decreases the amount of hematogenous and lymphatic seeding, thereby lowering recurrence rates [12]. Lasers have been employed for therapeutic as well as preventive for progression to malignancy in many such lesions like *leukoplakia, actinic chelitis, oral lichen planus* and *erythroplakia* and serve as a new minimally invasive and patient amenable modality. Lasers have also enabled optical biopsy. They are also referred to as *modern-day photoknife* [10, 12].

10.2. Lasers in Oral Leukoplakia

'Oral leukoplakia is a predominantly white lesion of the oral mucosa that cannot be characterized as any other definable lesion' (Axell et al., 1996). It is usually asymptomatic but may be associated with some degree of discomfort, including sensitivity to spicy or acidic foods. The prevalence of OL worldwide is ~2% (Petti, 2003), with a frequency greater in smokers than in non-smokers. Clinical features make its diagnosis, and a biopsy is mandatory to exclude other diseases. OL is a white plaque and is divided into homogeneous and non-homogeneous types: the homogeneous type is a white plaque that is flat, thin, and uniform, whereas the non-homogeneous type, can be irregularly flat, nodular, verrucous, and with a white and red colouration (van der Waal, 2010). With respect to non-homogeneous OL, proliferative verrucous leukoplakia (PVL) can involve any site in the oral cavity and has a high risk of malignant transformation (van der Waal and Reichart, 2008). A histological examination must be performed to exclude other diseases, and in particular, to determine the presence of dysplasia (mild, moderate, or severe; low-grade intraepithelial lesion or high-grade intraepithelial lesion, according to the 2014 Ljubljana classification). Malignant transformation ranged from 0.13% to 17.55% (Lee et al., 2006; Reibel, 2003). Thus, not all OL cases transform into OSCC. A high risk of malignant transformation is correlated with the degree of histological dysplasia.

Several treatment options have been used for OL, but, according to the literature, cold knife surgery and carbon dioxide (CO_2) laser surgery seem to offer better outcomes than topical or systemic medication in terms of recurrence and malignant transformation. Although there is no evidence that treatment prevents malignant transformation, it is recommended to treat OL with or without dysplasia (Horch et al., 1986; Chandu et al., 2005; Brouns et al., 2014a). Patel (1964) invented the CO_2 laser in 1963, but Ben-Bassat and coworkers (1978) were the first to describe its use for intraoral treatment. Usually, the laser of choice for oral leukoplakia treatment is the CO_2 laser as it is efficient in cutting oral soft tissues and only produces superficial thermal damage, resulting from the intense energy absorption of this particular wavelength (10,600 nm) by its main chromophores, water, found in abundance in the oral mucosa. Whenever oral leukoplakia is distributed in areas that are difficult to access with the CO_2 articulated arm, a laser with a flexible optical fibre, such as the diode laser (808–980 nm), can be used in a contact mode. Lasers have certain advantages over the scalpel and cryoprobe, in the management of oral leukoplakia, especially where large areas of epithelium are involved [10-12].

10.2.1. Lasers-Assisted Excision versus Scalpel Excision

A. Advantages of excision of oral leukoplakia by high power lasers over conventional method (i.e., scalpel) include: [12, 133, 134]

1. Bleeding control: laser surgery has a haemostatic effect, so it is very suitable for the surgical treatment of oral mucosal diseases, although the oral mucosa is rich with blood vessels.
2. The surgeon has improved visibility during the operation.

3. Less bacteremia.
4. Can be a particularly favourable technique when large areas of the oral mucosa are affected, as wound healing occurs by secondary intention.
5. Little collagen is deposited during healing and there is minimal interference with normal oral function. Keeps functional disorders to a minimum, because regeneration can occur without leaving postoperative cicatricial contractures.
6. Histologically, there are few myofibroblasts present, which appear to be responsible for less scar contraction.
7. Laser vaporization can be repeatedly performed under local anaesthesia on an outpatient basis, even if a new lesion occurs adjacent to the primary lesion.
8. The recurrence rate is low.
9. Reduced postoperative pain, swelling, oedema, or infection.
10. Sterile surgical field based on instant vaporization of tissue and adjacent vascular and lymphatic sealing.
11. It helps in preventing the seeding of the dysplastic cells in adjacent soft tissue areas.

B. Laser surgery has some disadvantages: [12, 133, 134]

1. The lesion is not available for histology, and this investigation is only done on small incisional biopsies. A biopsy must be obtained by other methods, either preoperatively or at the time of treatment, with laser vaporization.
2. Epithelial regeneration is delayed and wounds take longer to re-epithelialize than following excision surgery with sutures; small granuloma may sometimes be formed on the wound surface during healing.
3. Safety precautions are mandatory like the use of eyeglasses is needed to protect both the patient and the operator.

10.2.1.1. Laser Irradiation Protocol: [10, 13]

1. Surgery is performed with the CO_2 laser (continuous mode, 10 600 nm, 5–10 W) or diode laser (GaAlAs, ZAP softlase; continuous mode, 808 nm, 2–3 W) under local anaesthesia.
2. Initially, lesions are outlined by vaporization, creating a margin that is 3 mm deep, with a distance of ~5 mm from the lesion border.
3. Following lesion demarcation, the margin is lifted with forceps, and excision is carried out by undercutting at a constant depth.
4. Laser excision specimens are submitted for histopathological analysis.
5. Since the surgical treatment does not preclude oral leukoplakia from transforming into cancer and does not avoid oral leukoplakia recurrences, a close follow-up must be carried out. There is no evidence of optimal intervals of follow-up after oral leukoplakia treatment. However, lifelong follow-up at intervals of 6 months for non-dysplastic oral leukoplakia and of 3 months for dysplastic oral leukoplakia has been suggested. Few studies report the follow-up of all patients every 3 months, regardless of the grade of dysplasia.

10.2.1.2. New Concepts for the Recurrence and New Occurrence of Oral Leukoplakia [135]

Frame et al. reported that the new epithelium that migrates from the periphery to cover the wound might originate from an area of potentially unstable mucosa and that this may explain, why new patches of leukoplakia develop adjacent to the margins of previously treated areas. Reports show that the probability of developing recurrences and new occurrences was 40% after 3 years and 23% within 1 year of surgery. Based on these findings, it is important to ascertain the border of the lesion, because each kind of laser used can irradiate to a sufficient depth of the oral mucosal epithelium. Histologically, removal of the mucosal epithelium through vaporization was achieved consistently with CO_2

laser therapy (Figure 14). It is strongly recommended that vital tissue staining, such as iodine or toluidine blue staining immediately preoperatively is necessary to reduce local recurrences and malignant transformation because multicentric or micro invasive cancers have often developed from oral leukoplakia.

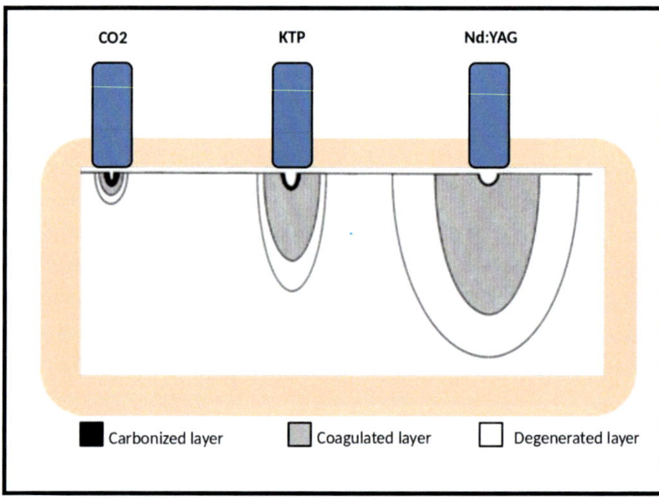

Figure 14. Comparison of the damage of soft tissue by CO_2, KTP and Nd: YAG laser.

A comparative collation of recent studies demonstrating the use of lasers in the treatment of oral leukoplakia has been summarized in Table 18.

10.3. Lasers in Actinic Chelitis

A comparative collation of recent studies demonstrating the use of lasers in the treatment of actinic chelitis using laser assisted excision/resurfacing and photodynamic therapy have been summarized in Table 19, 20, 21.

10.3.1. Laser-Assisted Excision and Resurfacing

While there is no consensus on surgical treatment of oral leukoplakia, excision of actinic cheilitis has been shown to be effective in preventing cancer progression. While oral leukoplakia is typically not associated with any aetiologic factor, except for tobacco, the aetiology of actinic cheilitis is known. UV light induces the occurrence of actinic keratosis in the skin of individuals excessively exposed to sunlight, especially those who are fair-skinned, and poses a risk to transformation in non-melanoma malignant neoplasia of the skin. This condition may affect the lips as well as the skin, involving predominantly the vermilion of the lower lip. Clinically, the appearance of actinic cheilitis of the lip is areas of dry, scaly patches and colour change. Atrophy, swelling, loss of vermilion margin, or ulceration correspond to signs of severe tissue damage, thus indicating the need for a biopsy. Actinic cheilitis may be successfully prevented with sunscreen lip balm, along with the recommendation to avoid sun exposure. However, if clinical changes on the lip are noted during follow-up and/or histopathological examination shows dysplasia, the use of topical agents (i.e., imiquimod, trichoroacetic acid or 5-fluorouracil), destruction (i.e., photodynamic therapy or cryosurgery) or removal of the tissue (by scalpel, electrodessication or high power laser) are treatment options that should be considered in order to avoid malignant progression [141]. Although vermilionectomy by scalpel is the gold standard treatment for actinic cheilitis, lip contour might be compromised, among other postoperative complications. The use of the CO_2 laser for surgical excision of the entire vermilion lip may be an alternative technique, with satisfactory wound repair and fewer adverse effects (less scarring and paresthesia), yet rendering tissue for histopathological analysis [11, 142].

Table 18. Use of Lasers in Oral Leukoplakia

Authors	Type of Study	Type of Laser	Laser Parameters	Results
Debanti Giri et al. (2016) [136]	Case Report	980 nm Diode laser	Continuous mode at 2 watts	On the 7th day follow-up, granulation tissue was seen which was the sign of secondary healing. The patient came after 11 and 13 days for follow-up. After 1 month, complete resolution of the lesion was seen without recurrence and restricted mouth opening.
Giacomo Del Corso et al. (2015) [137]	Retrospective study	Group 1: Nd:YAG laser Group 2:CO_2 laser	Group-1: 9 W for the lip, tongue, and marginal gingiva, and at 12 W for the remaining areas, pulsed mode, 3200 W/cm^2 to 4200 W/cm2, 3 to 10. Group 1- 8-15W, and used in pulse mode, 20 Hz, 10 to15 min.	No significant difference was found between the two treatments. However, CO_2 laser excision resulted in better results than the Nd:YAG laser evaporation, considering the non-homogeneous OLs and OLs with mild dysplasia.
Nita Chainani-Wu et al. (2015) [138]	Retrospective cohort study	CO_2 laser	wavelength 10.6 mm	This study has identified poor accessibility of the lesion margins as a predictor for early recurrence of leukoplakia following laser removal. Other variables evaluated did not reach statistical significance, possibly due to lack of power.
Pía López-Jornet et al. (2013) [139]	Prospective Study	CO_2 laser	continuous mode, defocalized, with 15 mm of distance focus-lesion, power setting of 5-15 W, 5-15 seconds	Pain and swelling reported by the patients were greater with the conventional cold knife than with the CO_2 laser, statistically significant differences for pain and swelling were observed between the two techniques during the first three days after surgery, followed by a gradual decrease over one week. In neither group was granuloma formation observed, and none of the patients showed malignant transformation during the period of follow-up.

Table 19. Laser-assisted excision and resurfacing in Actinic Chelitis

Authors	Type of Study	Type of Laser	Laser Parameters	Results
Cohen JL (2013) [142]	Interventional study	Erbium laser	2940 erbium laser	The author finds this modality useful for biopsy-proven AC, resurfacing of entire lip following complete SCC excision, and clinically prominent AC. Good overall results in AC due to ease of use, overall safety, tolerability, cosmetic acceptability.
Paul Armenores et al. (2010) [140]	Retrospective, interventional, nonrandomized, sequential case series	Er:YAG laser	Ablative pass (1 J/cm^2, variable pulse width; calculated by the efficiency of the laser head but reached up to 400 microseconds) or Coagulation pass (1 J/cm^2, with pulse width between 2 and 35 milliseconds)	"cure" rate of 84.8%, 5.1% experienced scarring, cosmetic benefit 68.8%, 0% functional worsening, 18.2% increased sensation, 2.6% decreased sensation.
IRIA Castiñeiras et al. (2009) [143]	Retrospective review	CO_2 laser system	Power density of 2 W/cm^2, using a focalized mode	3/43 had local recurrence of the AC, which occurred 16, 14, and 13 months after the treatment; improved after a new CO_2 laser treatment with total resolution. 2 had a minimal residual persistent scar without interference in the normal lip function. Overall, well-tolerated, cosmetic results satisfactory, excellent patient acceptance. 4.6% went on to develop lip SCC. The follow-up of these patients is mandatory.
Flávio Francisco de Godoy Peres et al. (2008) [141]	Prospective interventional comparative study	CO_2 laser	Group-A: Pulse energy of 350 mJ, at 3.5 W, amplitude 0.1, repetition rate of 6.6 Hz. Group B: pulse energy of 250 mJ , at 5W, with an amplitude of 0.05 s and a repetition rate of 10 Hz.	Re-epithelialization time following the 250-mJ protocol had mean 13.5 ± 3.34 days and 17.2 5 ± 3.77 days for 350-mJ. 1 patient showed peri-labial outbreak of herpes simplex 3 days after the procedure. The post-operative rate of AC lesions corresponded to 12.5% for each protocol. A reduction in the intensity of epithelial dysplasia was observed in the patients grouped according to the degree of dysplasia (absent, mild, moderate, and severe dysplasia) in the preoperative and postoperative period of both protocols.

10.3.2. Laser-Assisted Photodynamic Therapy

Photosensitizer: Methyl 5-aminolevulinate (MAL)

Table 20. Laser PDT in Actinic Chelitis using MAL

Authors	Type of Laser	Treatment Regimen	Results
Calzavara-Pinton et al. (2013) [144]	Red light	2.3 treatments at mean 9.6- day interval. Incubation: 3–4 hours; Dose: 37 J/cm^2.	CR of 27/43 (63%) at mean 4.2-month follow-up; other: 27/27 (100%) excellent cosmetic outcome in CR subjects.
Ribeiro et al. (2012) [145]	Red light, 630 nm	Incubation: 3 hours. Dose: 37 J/cm^2; Irradiance: 71 mW/cm^2; Time: 8 minute 40 seconds; Distance: 5–7 cm.	3/19 (16%) at mean 1.5-month follow-up; other: 80% clinical improvement judged by subjects, 80% mean subject satisfaction, level of dysplasia significantly decreased.
Fai et al. (2012) [146]	Red light, 630 nm	1–2 treatments at a 1-week interval. Incubation: 2–3 hours; Dose: 37 J/cm^2.	CR: 20/29 (69%) at mean 20-month follow-up; other: cosmetic outcome rated good to excellent in 97% of subjects.
Sotiriou et al. (2010) [147]	Red light 570–670 nm	Treatments at 2-week intervals, then, 4 weeks of imiquimod 5%. Incubation: 3 hour; Dose: 40J/cm^2; Irradiance: 80 mW/cm^2	CR: 24/34 (71%); HC: 22/34 (65%) at 12 month follow-up.
Castano et al. (2009) [148]	Red light 630 nm	1–3 treatments at 4-week intervals. Incubation: 3 hours; Dose: 50–80 J/cm^2.	CR: 3/3 (100%) at 3- to 6-month follow-up.
Rossi et al. (2008) [149]	Red light 630 nm	Treatments at 2-week interval. Incubation: 3 hours; Dose: 37 J/cm^2; Irradiance: 70–100 mW/cm^2; Time: 8 minutes 40 seconds.	CR: 5/5 (100%) at 30- month follow-up other: 5/5 (100%) with excellent cosmetic outcome.

Photosensitizer: 5-aminolevulinic acid (ALA)

Table 21. Laser PDT in Actinic Chelitis using ALA

Authors	Type of Laser	Treatment Regimen	Results
Zaiac and Clement et al. (2011) [150]	Blue light 417 nm	2 treatments at 3- to 5- week interval Incubation: 1–1.5 hours; time: 16 minutes 40 seconds	CR: 19% at 3- month follow-up; other: >75% clearance and excellent cosmetic outcomes in all subjects.
Sotiriou et al. (2008) [151]	Red light 570–670 nm	2 treatments at 2-week interval Incubation: 3 hours; dose: 40 J/cm^2; irradiance: 80 mW/cm^2	CR: 55%; HC: 43% at 18-month follow-up; other: 95% with good to excellent cosmetic outcome.
Alexiades-Armenakas and Geronemus et al. (2004) [152]	Long-pulsed dye laser 595 nm	1–3 treatments at 1 month intervals; 1 treatment with LP PDL in 2 control subjects Incubation: 2–3 hours; dose: 7.5 J/cm2; time: <1 minute 10 ms pulse, 10-mm spot size, 30 ms cryogen spray, 30 ms delay (2–3 passes)	CR: 13/19 (68%) at mean 4.1-month follow-up; no clinical response in 2 control subjects at 1-month follow-up.

10.4. LASERS IN ORAL ERYTHROPLAKIA

Erythroplakia very rarely affects the oral mucosa. According to large surveys of the general population, the prevalence of oral erythroplakia ranges from 0.02% to 0.13%. Clinically, oral erythroplakia usually presents as a (bright) red plaque, with signs of atrophy but no specific histopathological features. In most cases (close to 100%), lesions show severe dysplasia or superficial oral squamous cell carcinoma. The differential diagnosis should include erosive and atrophic oral lichen planus, and erythematous candidosis. The histopathological analysis helps the diagnosis by excluding lesions that have specific histopathological features [10].

Laser therapy offers a promising route for the treatment of oral erythroplakia (Table 22, 23). The carbon dioxide (CO_2) laser is a viable option, effectively vaporizing affected areas, followed by the removal of the heat-separated tissue. The CO_2 laser is potentially advantageous due to its precisely controlled thermal damage, with minimal effects on the tissue surrounding the target area. The neodymium-doped yttrium aluminum garnet (Nd:YAG) laser, which penetrates the skin to cause coagulation at a depth of 3–10 mm, has also been shown to effectively treat EOQ lesions. Additionally, photodynamic therapy (PDT) has also been used to treat basal cell carcinomas, SCC, and other skin cancers. Use of a photosensitizer, such as 5-aminolevulinic acid (ALA) or 5-methylaminolevulinic acid (MAL), causes an accumulation of protoporphyrin IX in tumour cells, which is subsequently activated by visible light. PDT causes selective destruction of abnormal cells with promising outcomes [10, 11].

10.4.1. Laser-Assisted Excision

Table 22. Use of laser excision for Erythroplakia

Authors	Type of Laser	Laser Parameters	Results
S. W. Yang et al. (2015) [154]	Carbon dioxide (CO_2) laser	power setting of 12–15 W in a continuous-wave mode	There was no postoperative malignant transformation, but invasive carcinoma found after initial excision (n = 3) was treated by further radical excision. The postoperative recurrence rate was 14/84 (16.7%).
Yamaguchi et al. (2014) [155]	CO_2 laser	Super-pulsed wave with surgical Excision; 10 W	Complete remission. No major complications or pain.
Losada et al. (2005) [156]	CO_2 laser	Continuous wave, 1 mm diameter, 5 W/Cm^2	Complete remission.

Authors	Type of Laser	Laser Parameters	Results
Conejo et al. (2005) [157]	CO_2	10,600 nm, 5 W, Super-pulsed wave	Relapse (N = 1, treated again with complete remission). Re-epithelialization at 14–28 days. Cosmetically excellent.
Bezooijen et al. (2001) [158]	Nd:YAG laser	23–30 W	Relapse in 14 %. Complete remission in (N = 7)
Bezooijen et al. (2001) [158]	CO_2 laser	15 W, Continuous wave, Repeated at 2–4 months	Relapse in 33 % (N = 4). Complete remission (N = 11).

10.4.2. Laser-Assisted Photodynamic Therapy

Table 23. Use of laser-PDT for Erythroplakia of skin and various mucosal surfaces

Authors	Type of Laser	Photo-sensitizer	Laser Parameters	Results
Cinotti et al. (2014) [159]	578 nm (copper bromide laser)	MAL	35 J/cm^2, 400 ms, ×2 at 2 weeks	CR at 5 months, determined by confocal technique. Confirmed at 1-year follow-up by skin biopsy.
Calzavara-Pinton et al. (2013) [160]	635 ± 18 nm	MAL	37 J/cm^2	CR (N = 5). Marked local reaction (N = 6), moderate (N = 1), no reaction (N = 1). Marked pain or burning during treatment (N = 3).
Park et al. (2012) [161]	Red light	MAL	37 J/cm^2 × 10 Over 4 months.	Decrease in size, but developed into invasive SCC. Partial penectomy resulted in Complete remission at 12 months. Tolerable discomfort during treatment.

Table 23. (Continued)

Authors	Type of Laser	Photo-sensitizer	Laser Parameters	Results
Fai et al. (2012) [162]	red light	MAL	37 J/cm^2, ×2 over 2 weeks.	CR (N = 19). Persistent lesion (N = 3). Persistent local symptoms delaying 2nd session by 1 week (N = 7). Pain, burning, erythema, edema, erosion/ulceration (N= 23). Blistering and dyschromia/ hyper pigmentation (N=4).
Paoli et al. (2006) [163]	600–730 nm	ALA+MAL	50–80 J/ cm^2, 35–80 mW/cm^2	Incomplete clearance (N = 1), Recurrence (N = 1). Pain and temporary superficial erosions. No scarring or deformities.
Wang et al. (2008) [164]	-	ALA	80–100 J/cm^2, 60 mW/cm^2	Complete remission (N = 6). Spread of lesion (N = 1). Minimal scarring.

10.5. Lasers in Oral Lichen Planus

Contrary to other OPMD's, the potential for malignant transformation of oral lichen planus is still controversial. Oral lichen planus is a polymorphous disease, with classification based on its varied clinical manifestations. The reticular and plaque-like, being the most common forms, affect about 60% of patients with oral lichen planus. These forms are symptomless, and do not require treatment but do require periodic evaluation. On the other hand, atrophic and erosive forms may be painful and require treatment. As a mainstream treatment, topical corticosteroids are widely used, although other therapies can also be used, such as topical retinoids. In some widely spread cases, short-term treatment with systemic corticosteroids may be necessary [10, 11].

Table 24. Use of LLLT in Oral Lichen Planus

Authors	Type of Study	Type of Laser	Laser Parameters	Results
Maria Mutafchieva et al. (2018) [166]	Interventional study	Diode laser, 810 nm	0.5 W, 30 s, 1.2 J/cm^2; Three times weekly for a month.	There was a significant reduction in pain after LLLT. Improvement in clinical signs was achieved in 59.3% of the lesions Complete resolution was revealed in 37.3% of the lesions. All patients experienced some degree of improvement. Most of the cases showed moderate recovery.
Wei-Bing Liu et al. (2017) [167]	Clinical study	Excimer laser, 308-nm	The initial dose was 250 mJ/cm^2, and gradually increased by 10–25 mJ/cm^2 each time according to the tolerance of patients, once per week.	The efficacy was satisfactory. The clinical symptoms of five patients were significantly improved. In two patients, the erosion surface completely disappeared, and clinical recovery was achieved. Three patients achieved partial remission. In the remaining one patient, the erosion surface had not completely healed. Only one patient had developed mild pain.
Zohaib Akram et al. (2017) [168]	Systematic review	Diode lasers (3 studies) In:Ga:Al:P (indium-gallium-aluminum-phosphate) laser (2 studies)	Laser wavelengths, power, spot size, and duration of laser exposure ranged between 630–970 nm, 10–3000 mW, 0.2-1.0 cm^2, and 6–480 s, respectively. The follow-up period ranged from 4 to 48 weeks.	All included studies reporting clinical scores showed that LLLT was effective in the treatment of OLP in adult patients at follow-up. Three studies showed significantly higher improvements with topical use of corticosteroids compared to LLLT, while one study showed significant improvement with LLLT. One study showed comparable outcomes between LLLT and corticosteroid application.

Table 24. (Continued)

Authors	Type of Study	Type of Laser	Laser Parameters	Results
Thomas Mücke et al. (2014) [169]	Clinical trial	CO_2 laser, 10.6 mm	Power output ranges from 1 to 20W and can be operated in a defocused continuous mode. A handpiece with a focal length of 125 mm was used. In focus, the spot has a diameter of 200 mm.	A total of 103 patients (60.2%) underwent symptomatic conservative treatment, and 68 patients (39.8%) underwent Continuous defocused CO_2 laser treatments. SCC developed in 16 patients (9.4%), 2 patients (2.9%) after continuous defocused CO2 laser treatment and 14 patients (13.6%) with symptomatic treatment only. This study provides insight into the potential impact of the CO_2 laser in the management of patients with erosive OLP and the influence on the recurrence rate of erosive OLP, as well as malignant transformation to oral SCC.
Adriana Cafaro et al. (2013) [170]	Prospective case series	Gallium-aluminum-arsenide (GaAIAs) diode laser, 980 nm	A collimated probe, a diameter of 0.6 cm and a spot size of 0.28 cm^2, was used. Power was 300 mW; Power density was 1 W/cm^2. A "spot" technique was used, covering all the mucosal lesions and the perilesional tissues up to 0.5cm. Fluence 4 J/cm^2 per lesion, the probe was held perpendicularly at a distance of about 2 mm.	79.27 % had symptom improvements already after the first four sessions of therapy. No reported complications or therapy side effects were observed in any of the patients treated.

Authors	Type of Study	Type of Laser	Laser Parameters	Results
F. Agha-Hosseini et al. (2012) [171]	Comparative study	CO_2 laser Diode laser (Ga–As)	Group A: CO_2 laser irradiation surgery at 10,600 nm, 3 W. Group B: Diode laser with two probes, infrared light (890 nm, 0.30.5J/cm^2) and red light (633 nm, CW, 0.3–0.5 J/cm^2). Each patient received light exposure for 5 sessions every other day.	After 3 months, the clinical response showed 100% and 85% partial to complete improvement in LLLT and CO_2 laser surgery, respectively. This demonstrates a quick and pronounced beneficial effect in controlling symptoms related to OLP. Both methods may be effective in the treatment of OLP and can be used as alternative therapy alongside standard treatment modalities.

Table 25. Use of PDT in Oral Lichen Planus

Authors	Type of Study	Type of Laser	Laser Parameters	Results
Sonja Radakovic et al. (2017) [172]	Clinical study	red light (RF-Rhodo LED, Biofrontera GmbH, Leverkusen, Germany)	630 ± 9 nm; The delivered light dose was 37 J/cm^2 at a light intensity of 61.7 mW/cm^2, illumination time was 10 minutes. The treatment routine included a second PDT session after two weeks.	Complete clinical response at the 3-month follow-up was achieved in 72.7%. Up to the final 12 months follow up, a recurrence was observed in two lesions. The complete clinical cure rate at 1 year after Alacare patch PDT thus was 66.6%. The cosmetic outcome of the treatment was excellent in all cases.
S. H. Choi et al. (2015) [173]	Prospective, randomized, comparative trial	Erbium:yttrium–aluminum–garnet ablative fractional laser-assisted methyl aminolaevulinate–PDT (Er:YAG AFL MAL-PDT, Joule; Sciton Inc., Palo Alto, CA, U.S.A)	A single session of Er:YAG AFL MAL PDT or two sessions of MAL-PDT. AFL therapy was performed using a 2940-nm Er:YAG AFL at 300-lm ablation depth, level 1 coagulation, 22% treatment density, and a single pulse For MAL PDT each treatment area was separately illuminated with red light-emitting diode lamps with peak emission at 632 nm and total light dose of 37 J cm^2.	Er:YAG AFL MAL-PDT was significantly more effective (92% complete response rate) than MAL-PDT (59%) at the 3-month follow-up, and differences in efficacy remained significant at the 12-month follow-up (85% in Er:YAG AFL MAL-PDT and 29% in MAL-PDT). The recurrence rate was significantly lower for Er:YAG AFL MAL-PDT (8%) than for MAL-PDT (50%) group at 12 months. No significant difference in cosmetic outcome or safety was observed between Er:YAG AFL MAL PDT and MAL-PDT.

Oral lichen planus can be difficult to treat and is sometimes refractory to conventional therapies. When the first-line approach is not producing any benefit, surgery may be performed. Some authors have reported that in recalcitrant or refractory cases of oral lichen planus, high power lasers should be considered as an option. As the CO_2 laser evaporation technique has been shown to be effective in the treatment of superficial mucosal lesions, it can also be applied to oral lichen planus lesions. Technical considerations may be the same for leukoplakia and actinic chelitis. However, instead of resecting the lesion, the laser beam swipes over the treatment area, penetrating to a depth of ~5 mm. In recent case reports, low power lasers (excimer, 308 nm; diode laser, 830 nm, 904 nm, and 630 nm) for recalcitrant cases of oral lichen planus have been shown to be effective for pain control. As of now, CO_2 vaporization or low power energy lasers have not been deemed as standard treatment modalities for oral lichen planus. Published reports suggest that low and high power lasers can be used as an option in cases non-responsive to conventional treatment (Table 24, 25) [10, 11].

Chapter 11

SURGICAL LASERS AND THEIR APPLICATIONS

11.1. INTRODUCTION TO LASERS IN ORAL SOFT TISSUE SURGERY

Before the advent of lasers, there were three main methods of oral surgical treatment available:

1. The conventional scalpel
2. Electro surgery
3. Cryotherapy (in use since the mid-1970s)

11.1.1. Basic Considerations for Choosing Laser as a Surgical Tool [10-12]

A. For the treatment of dental hard tissue, there are only a few wavelengths that may be used (Er:YAG, Er, Cr:YSGG, and CO_2). However, in soft tissue surgery, up to ten different wavelengths are applicable. The surgeon has a choice of a fibre-based delivery system

(Nd:YAG, diode lasers) or a non-contact optical system (CO_2, erbium family).

1. Diode lasers (445–1064 nm) are best used on pigmented tissue. They are small, compact instruments whose portability can be an advantage for short procedures. They are delivered through a small-diameter flexible optical fibre with an optional tip that can access small areas of tissue. Using a gated mode with digitally modulated pulse width and high-output-power diode laser has become very much more efficient than the early generations.
2. Nd:YAG (1064 nm) has a similar interaction with soft tissue although the free-running pulse mode can produce very high peak powers for efficiency. Its delivery system is the same as the diode.
3. KTP laser (532 nm) can be used similar to diode and Nd:YAG laser.
4. Ho:YAG laser (2100 nm) is mostly used in soft tissue surgery. It utilizes an articulated delivery system and noncontact application.
5. Argon laser (488, 514 nm) has its indications in the use for pigmented lesions or vascular malformations.
6. Carbon dioxide lasers (9300 and 10,600 nm) have been used traditionally in oral surgery, the latter wavelength having a very long history of clinical success. Higher average power than diode is readily available with very rapid tissue cutting speed, but there is a possibility of more tissue carbonization when used in continuous waves. Noncontact mode and the use of an articulated arm make the application more demanding.
7. Er:YAG (2940 nm) and the Er, Cr:YSGG(2780 nm) lasers are readily absorbed in water. Their main indication is hard tissue (bone) surgery. Soft tissue surgery is also possible but much slower. Haemostasis is not as prominent due to poor absorption in pigmented chromophores. Depending on the particular laser,

there is a choice of either contact or noncontact mode with the tissue, using delivery tips or a tip less hand piece.

B. The Shallow or Deeply Penetrating Lasers and Haemostasis [11]

The soft tissue lasers can be categorized into two broadly acting types: the deeply penetrating-type lasers (visible and near-infrared spectrum, 532–1,100 nm) that are essentially transmitted through water, showing a lower absorption coefficient in water such as KTP green laser. This explains their deep penetration into healthy soft tissue, such as Nd:YAG and diode lasers, in which the laser light penetrates and scatters deeply into tissue. However, they are selectively absorbed in areas of inflammation by blood components and tissue pigment. There is also minimal to no interaction of Nd:YAG and diode lasers with healthy (not covered by calculus) dental hard tissue, which makes them suitable for soft tissue procedures. The second category highlights the superficially absorbed lasers (CO_2, Er:YAG and Er,Cr:YSGG lasers), in which the laser beam is absorbed in the superficial layer and does not penetrate or scatter deeply. These lasers have a higher absorption coefficient in water, and due to the high water content of oral mucosa (>90%), they are very effective soft tissue lasers. The cost is relatively high and there are portability and movement issues.

1(a) The Nd:YAG laser is often used in free-running pulsed mode, with very short-duration pulses and an emission cycle (ratio of "on" time to total treatment time) of <1% and very high peak power per pulse (100–1,000 W).

1(b) The Nd:YAG laser is a deeply penetrating type of laser and produces a relatively thick coagulation layer on the lased soft tissue surface, exhibiting strong haemostasis. Therefore, the Nd:YAG laser is effective for the ablation of potentially haemorrhagic soft tissue.

1(c) Diode lasers represent a shallower penetration depth compared to Nd:YAG lasers and are less likely to cause pulpal damage after use. The diode lasers can be used in a continuous-wave or gated-CW mode and are the ideal choice for use in orthodontic set-up because of the smaller size ("footprint") of the laser device and relatively lower cost.

2(a) Soft tissue penetration depth for CO_2 laser is approximately 0.2 mm and for erbium lasers (Er:YAG and Er,Cr:YSGG lasers) can be as shallow as 5 μm.

2(b) CO_2 lasers have the highest absorption in hydroxyapatite and calcium phosphate and must be used with care during soft tissue procedures to avoid direct contact with hard tissue.

2(c) The CO_2 laser beam is absorbed in the tissue surface with very little scatter or penetration and is associated with a relatively thin layer of coagulation around the ablated site. The ablation for CO2 laser is basically caused by heat generation (carbonization).

2(d) Erbium lasers have the highest absorption into the water and target molecular water or the hydroxide ion as primary targets and mineral as a secondary target and therefore are used for ablation of both hard and soft tissues.

2(e) Erbium lasers provide the most rapid, favourable, and uneventful wound healing due to their precise ablation with minimal thermal effects as well as low inflammatory response.

2(f) However, haemostasis is less effective with the erbium lasers because of the minimal tissue denaturation, which guarantees subsequent sufficient bleeding and blood clot formation in the ablated defects and thereby induces favourable wound healing.

2(g) Overall, erbium lasers provide the highest absorption into the water, minimizing the thermal effects on the surrounding tissues during irradiation, but the cost, laser portability, movement, and less clear-cut incision morphology compared to CO_2 and diode lasers are the potential drawbacks.

C. Tissue Ablation: Non-contact or Contact Cutting Mode [11, 12]

Three forms of energy transfer can be observed:

- Radiation: Where the photon stream is delivered through a short airspace with no contact between delivery tip and target tissue. This may be commonly referred to as a "non-contact mode."

- Conduction: Where enhancement of the energy conversion can be achieved through direct contact between the delivery tip and the tissue. This may be commonly referred to as a "contact mode."
- Convection: Transfer of energy within the body of the tissue through fluid movement or circulation. This may occur regardless of either contact or non-contact modes.

Most surgical lasers produce a photothermal effect on soft tissue, evaporating soft tissues through the rapid thermal rise. The non-contact lasers such as CO_2 or erbium lasers (Er:YAG and Er,Cr:YSGG) directly and easily evaporate soft tissues by photothermal effects that vaporize interstitial water. However, the non-contact mode is associated with less precise cut and a lack of proprioceptive feedback compared to contact mode lasers. When lasers are used in contact mode to make an incision or excise soft tissue, they often need "initiation" of the laser tip end. In this process, part of the emitting light in the Nd:YAG and diode lasers is converted into heat by refraction or diffused reflection at the tip end, or in simple terms, the laser tip end gets initiated, creating a condition called "hot tip." This initiation produces secondary thermal effects at the heated tip end that can cut or incise soft tissue as well as offer coagulation of the tissue because of the contact with the overheated tip rather than by the laser energy itself.

11.1.2. Scalpel versus Lasers

1. Precision and visibility, haemostasis: Compared to conventional scalpel surgery, the diode laser cut is more precise and more visible due to the laser's ability to seal off blood vessels and lymphatics, leaving a clear dry field.
2. Surgical field sterilization: The laser also contributes to significant pathogen reduction as it cuts, and residual bacteria are evaporated, destroyed, or denatured by laser irradiation.

3. Combined effect: Laser incision with high-level laser therapy (HLLT) excises (ablates) the diseased tissues, with simultaneous provision of low-level laser therapy (LLLT) that penetrates or scatters into the surrounding tissues during high-level laser treatment and stimulates tissues and cells without producing irreversible changes.
4. Photobiomodulation with improved wound healing (Table 26), wound stabilization, less wound contraction, pain reduction, less need of local anaesthetic, bone repair and remodelling, nerve repair, and reduced oedema: PBM of tissues and cells following laser irradiation. LLLT generates an array of extremely transient biochemical intermediates that result in cascading biological reactions in favour of tissue healing. This process works by altering the cellular redox state and production of reactive oxygen species (ROS) in mitochondria, such as superoxide and hydrogen peroxide, which mainly affect and stimulate cells in a low redox state. Cells in a low redox state are acidic, but after laser irradiation, the cells become more alkaline and are able to perform optimally, inducing the activation of numerous intracellular signalling pathways [10-12].
5. Aesthetics: The use of adequate energy for cutting will produce little carbonization, leaving the wound unchanged in colour and structure. This makes orientation during the procedures easier, even for the surgically inexperienced dentist. When using the laser, not only is the wavelength important but also parameters like temporal emission mode (continuous wave or pulsed), pulse duration, emission cycle, exposure time, and the speed of the incision. All this, in the right proportions, will lead to a clean cut with little carbonization and contraction of proteins resulting in scarring.

Hence, compared with a scalpel, a laser beam or the initiated fiber-optic tip of the laser device can more easily cut, ablate, and reshape the oral soft tissues in the oral cavity, with no or reduced bleeding and less pain, as well as with no or less need for suturing. This represents a range of tissue interactions, such as tissue warming, welding, coagulation, protein, denaturation, drying, and finally vaporization (ablation), and carbonization, where soft tissues are evaporated or incised. This process also provides haemostasis, microbial inhibition, destruction, and photobiomodulation (PBM). In particular, there is increasing evidence that the appropriate use of lasers is associated with reduced intraoperative and post-operative pain and enhanced wound healing or tissue regeneration, compared to the conventional use of scalpel or electro surgery. Electro surgery can be used for incising soft tissues with good haemostasis, but comes with a risk of delayed wound healing due to unwanted thermal damage and necrosis of the underlying periosteum and alveolar bone.

Table 26. Effects of photobiomodulation (PBM) on four phases of wound healing [11]

Hemostatic phase	Promotes platelet aggregation and activation
Inflammatory phase	Promotes proliferation and degranulation of mast cells
Proliferative phase	Promotes proliferation of fibroblasts, keratinocytes, osteoblasts, and chondrocytes as well as induces matrix synthesis
Maturation phase	Improves reorganisation and remodelling of wounds, aids improved tensile strength and restores functional architecture of the repaired tissues

The various lesions, which can be treated using lasers, include:

1. Oral papillomas
2. Fibromas
3. Lipomas
4. Inflammatory fibrous and papillary hyperplasias
5. Drug-induced gingival overgrowth
6. Pyogenic granuloma
7. Peripheral giant cell granuloma and peripheral ossifying fibroma
8. Oral mucocele

9. Sialolithiasis
10. Haemangiomas, lymphangiomas, vascular malformations

11.2. Lasers in Oral Fibromas

The lesion most commonly found in the oral cavity is the fibroma. It occurs as a discrete, superficial, pedunculated mass commonly found on the buccal mucosa. It is usually of non-neoplastic nature and arises as a response to mechanical, chemical, and inflammatory agents. It is composed of collagenous, fibrous connective tissue covered with keratinized or parakeratinized squamous epithelium. In the lesion, there can be myxomatous degeneration or pathological weakening of the connective tissue along with bone formation and growth of fatty tissue. The patients often notice the lesion only after masticating on the area and then experiencing post-traumatic pain and swelling. At this point, the fibroma will have grown to at least 2–3 mm in size depending on the region and would be visible in a mirror [10, 11].

When a scalpel is used, postoperative bleeding often makes the procedure difficult, especially if the lesion is inflamed with increased vascularization. Moreover, suturing is often necessary. Laser surgery allows both excision and haemostasis simultaneously. The wound is normally left open for free secondary granulation. Consequently, laser surgery incurs minimal morbidity and promotes a more conservative surgery, greater haemostasis control, and reduced clinical time. In addition, precise dissection of tissue allows for adequate microscopic analysis of the specimen and makes the laser an adequate tool for diagnosis and treatment [10, 11, 174].

On the other hand, delayed repair and tissue necrosis may be observed even when adequate parameters are applied. Any temperature higher than 100°C results in volatilization of the tissue, smoke formation, and potential tissue damage. Therefore, the use of high-power lasers requires appropriate training for good clinical results and reduced risk of irreversible tissue damage. Postoperative complications such as pain, bleeding, difficulties with speech, obstructive submandibular sialadenitis, and paraesthesia of the lingual nerve have been reported after laser surgical treatment of potentially malignant lesions. An extremely rare, but reported complication is airway fire during the operation.

Vescovi et al. evaluated the impact of the laser-associated thermal effect on the histopathological features of fibrous hyperplasia removed with an Nd:YAG laser. It was demonstrated that lesions with a diameter of less than 7 mm suffer serious thermal effects, regardless of the parameters used, but these do not impair microscopic diagnosis. While the microscopic diagnosis of FH is sound and clear, the diagnosis of other lesions with more complex histopathological features or the grading of epithelial dysplasias may be impaired following their morphological alteration with laser surgery. To avoid compromising the biopsy of small lesions for diagnostic purposes, it can be recommended that laser surgery be only indicated for the biopsy of lesions larger than 1 cm. [10, 11, 12, 174].

11.3. Lasers in Oral Papillomas

Oral squamous papilloma (OSP) is benign epithelial neoplasia associated with the proliferation of the oral epithelium, which promotes a papillary or verrucous surface associated with human papilloma virus (HPV) infection. HPV is a large family of more than 100 subtypes of double-stranded DNA viruses with a remarkable affinity for epithelial cells. Some subtypes of HPV are associated with benign lesions of the oral cavity, and subtypes 6 and 11 are associated with OSP. Verruca vulgaris, condyloma acuminatum, and multifocal epithelial hyperplasia (Heck's disease) are examples of benign lesions associated with other subtypes of HPV. OSP is clinically characterized as a painless, non-bleeding, pedunculated, exophytic lesion with a verrucous surface forming a cauliflower-like aspect, and microscopically characterized by finger-shaped epithelial projections [10, 12].

Oral lesions occur mostly on the tongue, lips, and soft palate, but any site can be affected. The lesions present no gender predilection and are found at any age, but more commonly in the fourth to fifth decades of life. OSP often presents as a single lesion with a white surface, but coalescent multiple lesions may occur (papillomatosis). Despite the distinctive clinical features, other verrucous or HPV-associated lesions, such as verruciform xanthoma, condyloma accuminatum, oral warts, and oral focal epithelial hyperplasia, should be considered in the differential diagnosis. Therefore, regardless of clinical presentation, biopsy followed by histopathological analysis should always be performed to confirm the diagnosis. Surgical removal of the lesion is an effective treatment, and recurrence is rarely observed. Laser surgery may also be a suitable treatment option for the management of OSP, reducing surgical time and postoperative complications [175, 176].

The laser removal of OSP is associated with tissue volatilization and the risk of HPV contamination. HPV DNA has been identified in the plume generated during CO_2 laser treatment of respiratory tract papillomas and plantar warts, but the fact whether or not these dispersed viral particles are infectious, remains elusive. Nevertheless, recurrent respiratory papillomatosis was reported in healthcare workers who performed repeated laser therapies for patients with genital warts. On the other hand, a recent study by Ilmarinen et al. showed that protective equipment, mostly surgical gloves, may become contaminated by HPV, but human viral transmission is unlikely if protective devices are properly used. Rigorous use of protective devices, including laser plume masks, saline irrigation to reduce plume production, and an effective surgical aspirator may diminish the risk of HPV contamination and are warranted for the safety of the patient and the dental team [10, 12, 176].

11.4. Lasers in Oral Lipomas

Lipomas are the most common benign tumours of the human body. They can be solitary or in multiple clusters. They vary highly in size from minute to large growths, with weight in the kilograms. They occur mostly between 40 and 50 years of age. In the oral cavity, they appear as soft, slightly elastic, and painless lesions and are usually noticed by the patients if they are a large dimension. They are normally found in the buccal, submandibular, and vestibular regions. The development of a lipoma is not necessarily hereditary although hereditary conditions, such as familial lipomatosis, can stimulate its growth [178]. Genetic studies support prior epidemiologic data in humans showing a correlation between high-mobility group proteins (HMG I-C) and mesenchymal tumours.

When the patient's complaint is the size of the lesion, or to verify the diagnosis, the treatment is excision. The laser's ability to achieve instant haemostasis offers a good view of the site, which is important in some areas of the mouth, for example, in direct proximity to the mental nerve. While any wavelength will perform the surgery, a fibre-delivered laser that has better manoeuvrability could be an advantage in the depth of the wound. Depending on the dimension of the lesion, sutures would be placed to avoid food impaction [11, 12].

11.5. Lasers in Oral Pyogenic Granulomas

Pyogenic granuloma (PG) is a vascular lesion of the skin and oropharyngeal mucosa. It appears, as a reddish overgrowth due to mechanical, physical, chemical, or hormonal trauma, is generally located in the anterior of the maxilla, and can be painful if it is constantly irritated. The lesion can grow rapidly and will often bleed profusely after little or no trauma, and it has the appearance of highly vascular granulation tissue with inflammation on histologic examination. Special variants of the pyogenic granuloma are the epulis granulomatosum and the granuloma gravidarum. Treatment is not necessary except in cases of excessive bleeding or pain and ulceration. After pregnancy, the lesion normally regresses. Recurrence is in the range of 8% for laser surgery and 15% for conventional treatment [179]. As expected, any surgical laser that achieves good control of bleeding may be used. A biopsy must be taken for histological verification of the lesion [10, 11].

Microscopic examination of PG shows a highly vascular proliferation that resembles granular tissue. Numerous vessels, small and larger endothelium-lined channels, are formed that are engorged with red blood cells. These vessels are sometimes organized in lobular aggregates. The surface is usually ulcerated and a thick fibrino-purulent membrane then replaces this. A mixed inflammatory cell infiltrate of neutrophils, plasma cells, and lymphocytes is evident. Neutrophils are most prevalent near the ulcerated surface; chronic inflammatory cells are found deeper in the specimen. Being a non-neoplastic growth, excisional therapy is the treatment of choice. Although the conventional treatment for PG is surgical excision, a recurrence rate of 16% has been reported. There are also reports of the lesion being excised with an electric scalpel or cryosurgery. Other reported methods include cauterization with silver nitrate, sclerotherapy with sodium tetradecyl sulfate and monoethanolamineoleate ligation, absolute ethanol injection dye, the Nd:YAG33 and CO_2 lasers, high-power diode laser shave excision, and laser photocoagulation [10, 11, 12].

11.6. Lasers in Oral Vascular Lesions

11.6.1. Lasers in Oral Haemangiomas

Over the last 35 years, the term haemangioma has evolved to describe any number of vasoformative tumours thanks to Mulliken and Glowacki [180] who produced the classification scheme that is generally accepted today. However, it is important to note that the different clinical entities named haemangioma have little in common other than the fact that they all involve blood vessels. The classification differentiates between the group of haemangiomas and other vascular malformations. Haemangiomas are tumours characterized by rapid endothelial cell proliferation in early infancy, followed by involution over time.

Everything else is a vascular malformation with a normal endothelial growth. A haemangioma develops in the first months after birth and subsequently grows rapidly. It usually regresses over time, and only 10% are treated in adolescence. Conversely, a vascular malformation, such as a venous lake, shows little to no regression and very slow, stable growth. It is treated when it becomes a functional impairment or for aesthetic reasons. These lesions can be excised conventionally, which easily produces a biopsy specimen. The main disadvantage of that procedure is that a defect and scarring can result, especially on the lip. An alternative technique is to use the laser in a non-contact mode, aiming the photonic energy at the lesion, starting on the circumference and working toward the centre, until there is blanching and induration of the malformation. There will be a tissue temperature rise during lasing to achieve coagulation, and, with careful technique, thermal damage to the surrounding structures could be minimal. One protocol employing the deeply penetrating diode or Nd:YAG wavelengths include the using of an ice cube to cool the tissue while lasing through the ice [181]. The postoperative outcome of the noncontact treatment of vascular malformations shows an extremely high success rate and little postoperative discomfort [10, 11, 12].

11.6.2. Lasers in Lymphangiomas

Lymphangioma, first described in 1828 by Redenbacher, is a relatively rare occurrence. De Serres et al. proposed a classification of the lymphangioma of the head and neck based on the spread of the anatomical involvement [182].

- Stage/Class I: Infrahyoid unilateral lesions
- Stage/Class II: Suprahyoid unilateral lesions
- Stage/Class III: Suprahyoid and infrahyoid unilateral lesions
- Stage/Class IV: Suprahyoid bilateral lesions
- Stage/Class V: Suprahyoid and infrahyoid bilateral lesions

Considered by many as a congenital malformation of the lymphatic system, others consider it a benign vascular tumour of the lymphatic system arising from the proliferation of lymph vessels or a congenital haematoma. It is histologically benign, but infiltrative features may expand into the surrounding tissue, causing complications. Most lymphangiomas are present at birth (60%), and by the age of 2 years, 80–90% is present. It usually occurs in the head and neck, followed by the extremities, trunk, and abdomen. In the head and neck area, the most common location is the submandibular region, followed by the parotid gland. When a lymphangioma occurs in the mouth, the anterior two-thirds of the tongue is the most commonly affected region. In the oral cavity, lymphangioma also may involve the palate, gingiva, buccal mucosa, lips, and alveolar ridge of the mandible. Lymphangioma persists throughout life with periods of a temporary decrease in total volume. The diagnosis of lymphangioma with superficial infiltration of skin and mucosa by vesicles is tomography, and magnetic resonance imaging may be used to detect the cystic component and low flow that characterizes the lymphangioma [10, 12].

Various methods have been tried in the treatment of lymphangioma, including surgery, conventional high power laser surgeries, radiation, laser therapy, and sclerotherapy. A more conservative surgical approach using radio frequency ablation has been described in a case of lymphangioma in the right buccal mucosa of the mental foramen area. Radio frequency ablation therapy has several advantages for patients with lymphatic malformations. First, the technique can target areas of tissue involvement, sparing critical anatomical neurovascular components and sensitive mucosal surfaces. Second, the treatment delivered is not limited by the diffusion of injected agents, as in sclerosing therapy (this appears to be a weakness in the use of OK-432). Third, the procedure entails minimal invasive techniques and avoids significant pain and morbidity. This new and effective technique offers a clear benefit over the alternative treatments [183].

Although surgical excision is considered as a mode of treatment by most surgeons, this can leave the patient with several morbid conditions, such as nerve injuries, prolonged lymphatic drainage from the wound, recurrent lesions, wound infections, unacceptable scar formation, and incomplete resection due to infiltration of adjacent vital structures. Boiling water, quinine, sodium morrhuate, urethane, iodine tincture, and nitromin have been used as sclerosing agents with low success rates and several side effects. Recently, some surgeons in the treatment of lymphangioma have favored two sclerosing agents, bleomycin, and OK-432, and α-interferon 2a. While complete surgical removal has been the treatment of preference, where there is infiltrative lymphangioma, this is difficult and only possible in 10–50% of cases. Because of this, the recurrence rate is a major problem: 0–27% after complete removal and 15–53% after partial removal. Surgery is indicated when lesions are resectable and it does not promote mutilation or sequelae [184]. Low-level laser therapy (LLLT) is a form of phototherapy that involves the application of a low-power laser to areas of the body in order to stimulate healing and reduce pain and inflammation. This therapy may be used to reduce tumour size and control pain and inflammation [10].

11.7. Lasers in Salivary Gland Pathosis

11.7.1. Lasers in Oral Mucocele

Several clinical reports have described protocols for the application of laser irradiation in the excision of oral mucoceles. The large majority have used high power CO_2 lasers for excision or vaporization of the lesions, with a power range from 4 to 10 W. Few studies have described the use of Nd:YAG, Er:Cr:YSGG, and diode lasers (Table 27) [10].

Clinical outcomes indicate some advantages of using laser irradiation over the conventional surgical technique:

1. Short time of surgery: the procedure of mucocele excision using a CO_2 laser is brief in comparison with that using a scalpel,

mainly because sutures are unnecessary. This aspect is important, particularly in paediatric patients [197]

2. Immediate haemostasis: during incision and vaporization of the salivary gland, there is no bleeding, which favours clear visualization of the lesion margins. Some reports have described additional CO_2 laser irradiation in defocused mode at conclusion of surgery, in order to increase haemostasis and shrinkage of the lesion [10, 197]
3. Minor postoperative complications: reported postoperative complications are restricted to prescription of analgesics for a few patients, and transitory local paresthesia at the operative site. Good healing, and no scar formation were frequently reported [197]

Table 27. Laser-based excision of oral mucoceles [10]

Author	Laser Protocols	Clinical Outcomes
Frame [198]	CO_2 laser, 10 W, cw or pw	Good healing
Jinbu et al. [199]	Nd:YAG laser, 10 W, cw	Complete vaporization of the lesions; No recurrence after 3 years
Kopp and St Hilaire [200]	CO_2 laser, 6–8 W, cw	Good healing after 1 week
Niccoli-Filho and Morosolli 201	CO_2 laser, 4 W, cw	Good healing; no recurrences after 6 months
Bornstein et al. [202]	CO_2 laser, 3–9 W, cw or sp	16.6% recurrences; Temporarily diminished sensation in the oral mucosa after the laser excision
Zola et al. [203]	Er,Cr:YSGG laser, 11% air, 7% water, 1.5 W	Good healing
Kato and Wijeyeweera [204]	CO_2 laser, 3–4 W, cw	11% experienced postoperative pain; Good healing
Huang et al. [205]	CO_2 laser, 5–8 W, cw	1.21% patients had transitory local paresthesia at the operative site; 2.43% recurrences after 3 months
Yagüe-García et al. [206]	CO_2 laser, 5–7 W, cw	Good healing
Boj et al. [207]	Er,Cr:YSGG laser, 0% air, 0% water, 0.25 W	No scar formation; No recurrences after 12 months
Pedron et al.208	Diode laser (810 nm), 2 W, cw, contact	No recurrences after 12 months

11.7.2. Lasers in Sialolithiasis

Sialolithiasis is the occurrence of a salivary stone or calculus and is a frequent cause of inflammatory changes within the large salivary glands. Statistics show that over 78% of salivary stone formation affects the submandibular gland and 81% appear in the parotid gland, but is a rare occurrence in the sublingual gland, though not totally unknown. Conventional instrumentation offers no control of bleeding, and with the flow of saliva, visibility can be extremely difficult during the surgery. A laser ensures good haemostasis and therefore a good overview of the operation site. Sutures are not usually placed, and the healing is uneventful with little scaring [10, 11].

Chapter 12

LASER DIAGNOSTICS

12.1. LASER IN CARIES DETECTION

12.1.1. Quantitative Light-Induced Fluorescence (QLF)

The use of *fluorescence* in caries detection was originally suggested more than a century ago; current optical caries detection techniques emerged with the introduction of laser technology. In the 1980s, a clinically applicable visual detection method focusing on the natural green fluorescence of tooth tissue was developed [10]. The technique used a 488-nm excitation wavelength from an argon-ion laser to discriminate bright-green–fluorescing healthy tooth tissue from poorly fluorescing carious lesions. This technique was further refined in the early 1990s; the argon-ion laser was replaced by a xenon-based arc lamp, with the emission light shining through a blue-transmitting filter. This became known as *quantitative light-induced fluorescence* (QLF), using the digitization of images to quantify the observed green-fluorescence loss as an indirect measure of mineral loss. QLF is a highly sensitive method for determining short-term changes in hard tissue lesions in the mouth. The excitation wavelength (~405 nm) produced by the QLF system allows visualization and quantification of both the intrinsic green fluorescence of dental tissue and the *red-fluorescence* of bacterial origin, as observed in calculus, plaque, and advanced caries. The green-fluorescence loss from de-mineralized enamel and natural carious lesions strongly correlates with mineral loss. The red fluorescence of bacteria allows identification of leaking margins of sealants and restorations [11]. The phenomenon of substantial red fluorescence using laser wavelengths between 650 and 800 nm in carious lesions, much brighter than that of sound enamel or dentin, has resulted in a hand-held device to detect dental caries. Kavo (Germany) manufactured the first such unit in 1998, with an emission wavelength of 655 nm. The accuracy of results in primary tooth enamel is a concern, possibly a result of the reduced mineral density. The presence of existing restorations (amalgam, gold, porcelain, composite) appears to allow the detection of only marginal caries. Differences between QLF and DIAGNOdent: QLF uses a much shorter wavelength at 488 nm and is designed to detect and receive 540 nm auto fluorescent light from the enamel (it filters out the shorter wavelength scattered light using a 520 nm filter) The DIAGNOdent uses a longer wavelength 655 nm light and measures fluorescence intensity (uses a 680 nm filter) [11, 12].

12.1.2. Fibre-Optic Transillumination (FOTI) and Digital Imaging Fibre-Optic Transillumination (DIFOTI)

These are Transillumination Techniques. DIFOTI uses high-intensity light from a fibre-optic device source to illuminate a tooth, and the backscattered light is captured by a digital camera and analysed by a computer. Carious enamel and dentin would scatter light more than sound tooth structure and appear darker This technique has the advantage that it precludes the use of ionizing X-radiation and also provides diagnosis in real-time, and studies have shown that DIFOTI has a higher sensitivity than conventional radiography. The technique relies heavily on the judgment of the practitioner and suffers from many variabilities. It also does not indicate lesion depth or severity [10].

12.1.3. Polarization-Sensitive Optical Coherence Tomography (PS-OCT)

These techniques have proved successful at imaging hard and soft tissue in the oral cavity, providing numerical analysis of the optical properties of the surface and subsurface enamel. At research levels, using a near-IR beam (λ 1310 nm), caries detection is possible at both surface level and under composite restorations and sealants. Other spectroscopic devices use Raman-effect phenomena to quantify mineral loss associated with dental caries [6, 10].

12.1.4. Laser-Induced Breakdown Spectroscopy (LIBS)

These work on the principle that a highly intense but very short laser pulses of ultraviolet (UV), visible or infrared range (IR) would ablate target tissue into an expanding plasma plume of electrons, ions, and atoms. This luminous plasma plume would emit characteristic qualitative and quantitative structural and molecular information about the tissue being examined. R. V. Ambartsumyan and N. G. Basov et al. Ca first suggested the creation of such plasma and the theoretical basis of its breakdown and Na spectral lines were observed in healthy and carious teeth. The spectra from carious tooth minerals were «weaker» (in intensity and line width) than those from healthy tooth structures. Samek et al. (2001) used a Q-switched Nd.YAG laser, 1064 nm at 20 Hz, 4–8 ns pulses, with pulse energy 10–30 mJ on 159 carious and healthy extracted teeth and even in vivo on the molar tooth of a volunteer. They confirmed that LIBS along with pattern recognition algorithms like discriminant analysis can positively identify between carious and healthy tooth structure, to a precision of 100–200 μ laterally and 10 μ in depth. They inferred that this is possible through analysis of the spectra of matrix elements such as Ca or P and non-matrix elements like Li, Sr, Ba, Na, Mg, Zn, and C using pattern recognition algorithms. They stated that in carious tooth structure there would be a decrease in matrix elements and an increase in non-matrix elements.

12.1.5. Raman Spectroscopy

It has varied noninvasive diagnostic applications for oral hard tissues. The precision of such techniques makes it invaluable in the early diagnosis of carious lesions. Tactile, visual, or radiographic detection, perhaps, is not until the carious lesion has considerably progressed with an accompanying quantum of mineral loss from the teeth whereas this diagnostic technique is even able to identify changes in crystallinity such as orientation and symmetry of crystals of the tooth structure. Raman spectroscopy has also found useful indications in the detection of fluorousis and manifestations of developmental disorders such as amelogenesis imperfecta and characterization of the mineral phases in calculus. The fluorophores that could be detected by Raman spectroscopy are produced by various groups of bacteria too; hence, detection of plaque or incipient carious lesions is also possible [11, 12].

12.2. Laser Doppler Flowmetry

Laser Doppler flowmetry (LDF), originally in development, termed as laser Doppler velocimetry, uses laser light (632, 780–820 nm) to measure pulpal blood flow and thus tooth vitality by measuring the backscatter (change in frequency or collimation) on the same principle of interferometry as used in OCT [210-213]. Laser Doppler flowmetry has a range of applications in dentistry, though chiefly in endodontics and paediatric dentistry (in assessing the pulpal vitality of traumatized or avulsed teeth and age-related changes in pulp [214] but also in other fields like in orthodontics (measuring pulpal blood flow during tooth movement and treatment such as rapid maxillary expansion (RME) [215], in maxillofacial surgery (to confirm the vitality of teeth after orthognathic surgery and revascularization of reimplanted teeth and even in implantology (as an aid in evaluating implant stability [216]. LDF may not be very effective in teeth with restorations, the signal being affected by adjacent tissues like periodontal tissues and requiring isolation of the teeth being examined by a rubber dam or cotton rolls. Variations between the anatomy and position of the tooth in the arch, the laser wavelength, frequency of bandwidth and filter, probe design, and fibre separation (250–500 μ) all can affect the reliability of LDF.

12.3. Optothermal Radiometry

Pulse laser heating of tissue causes temperature perturbations and the corresponding modulation of its thermal (infrared) radiation. This is the basis for pulse optothermal radiometry (OTR). The significance to dentistry of this technique is caused by its potentiality to monitor dental lesions at the early stages of carious decay, where lateral and subsurface spatial resolution in the order of the crack sizes and subsurface depths. In dental practice, it is often desirable to obtain detailed local information on potential lesions, and inside pits and fissures with high spatial resolution, such as that achieved with a focused laser source. To meet these objectives, recently, a combination of FD-OTR and FD-LUM (luminescence) was used as a fast dental diagnostic tool to quantify sound enamel or dentin as well as subsurface cracks in human teeth [6].

12.4. Optical Coherence Tomography

Optical coherence tomography (OCT), a modality adopted from ophthalmology (Naohiro Tanno, David Huang 1991) is a noninvasive, live, imaging technique that provides three-dimensional high-resolution (10–15 μ) images to a depth of ~2 mm. Literally, it allows the diagnosis of pathology in tissues by optical methods without actually physically harvesting it from a patient surgically. It is based on the principle of backscattered light analysed through low-coherence interferometry, which in simple terms means that the light scattering back off a surface is superimposed (as constructive interference and destructive interference) to develop useful diagnostic data. The backscattered (reflected) light from the substrate generates a low coherence beam from differing depth levels (depending on tissue structures in the volume being imaged) to the interferometer. The optical data from each single scan point is interpreted by the interferometer as an interference pattern and recorded as a depth profile (A-scan), whereas a linear scan across the sample delivers cross-sectional (B-scan) data. The images can be based on spectral-domain scans of a single focus or swept laser light sources where the light of varying frequencies can be emitted sequentially [10-12].

12.4.1. Principle of OCT [217-219]

The functional principle behind OCT imaging is light interference, with a light interference setup being the core. In an OCT system, the light from a low-coherence source is split into two paths by a coupler directing it along two different arms of an interferometer. One arm is designated as the reference arm, while the other is the sample arm. When the light exits the fibre end of either arm, it is shaped by various optical components (mirrors, lenses, etc.) to control specific beam parameters such as shape, depth of focus, and the intensity distribution of the light. In the reference arm, the light is back reflected by a reference mirror, and it returns into the interference system, propagating along the same path it came from but in the opposite direction. The same process happens with the light in the sample arm, the only difference being that the beam is backscattered by the sample. In an inhomogeneous sample, different structures within the sample will have different indices of refraction and light will be backscattered when it encounters an interface between materials of different refractive indexes. The returning light from both arms recombine at the coupler and generates an interference pattern, which is recorded by the detector. For a particular position of the reference mirror, the light propagating in the reference arm travels a certain optical distance and forms the corresponding interference pattern only with the light that travelled the same optical distance along the sample arm, including the portion of the distance travelled inside the sample. Therefore, when the reference mirror is translated along the propagation direction of light, for different positions of the mirror, the returning reference generates interference patterns with light backscattered from corresponding depths within the sample. In this way, the dependence on the depth of the intensity of light backscattered from beneath the sample surface can be measured. The OCT signal recorded by the detector during a complete travel of the reference mirror is called a depth scan or an A-scan. In order to form an OCT image, the sample beam has to be translated across the sample surface, with an A-scan being recorded at each position of the beam. Therefore, a set of consecutive A-scans is obtained, forming an OCT image or otherwise called a B-scan.

12.4.1.1. Different Versions of Optical Coherence Tomography

12.4.1.1.1. Time-Domain (TD)-OCT

First or the original version is time-domain (TD)-OCT in which the position of reference mirror is changeable, and this property helps to detect the backscattered tissue intensity levels from different depths in a tissue sample. This prototype allows for obtaining images in both axial or A-scan (depth of penetration) and lateral or angular axis. TD-OCT works at a speed of 400 axial scans per second. Advancements in the basic version are mainly aimed at increasing the scanning speed with better axial resolution [217, 219].

12.4.1.1.2. Fourier Domain Optical Coherence Tomography

It is so named because it makes use of intensity profiles (A-scans) obtained by using a Fourier transform of the detected frequencies. This type further includes spectral-domain (SD)-OCT and swept-sources

(SS)-OCT. SD-OCT makes use of a broadband light source with a stationary reference mirror and the intensity of backscattered light is split by grating into frequency components which is detected by a charge-coupled device (CCD) that helps in improvising the resolution of axial scans. SD-OCT works at a speed of 312,500 axial scans per second. SS-OCT is a combination of both TD-OCT and SD-OCT in which the light source is a single tunable laser but not broadband light as in SD-OCT, also the CCD is replaced by a single photo detector. This modification resulted in improved transverse resolution and is mainly useful for visualizing finer transverse details like imaging of axons and blood vessels. SS-OCT works at a speed of 249,000 axial scans per second [217-219].

12.4.1.1.3. Polarization Sensitive Optical Coherence Tomography

Polarization sensitive OCT is another functional variant that uses polarization properties of light for imaging. Usually, light travels in the form of an electromagnetic wave in which the electric and magnetic fields are orthogonal to its propagation direction. Light wave is said to be linear polarized when all its electric field vectors are in a straight line during its propagation. Light tissue interactions alter this polarization of light, and recording this alteration will help in knowing both structural and functional abnormalities for a given tissue specimen. In order to achieve this, a polarizer first polarizes light emitted from the source before it passes through the beam splitter. A quarter-wave plate is added near the reference mirror that aids in confirming the polarized nature of the reference beam, and an additional polarized beam splitter near detectors that directs the resultant light toward the horizontal and vertical detectors. It is mainly used for imaging neoplasms, teeth defects, and collagen alterations in tissues [217, 219].

12.4.1.1.4. Doppler Optical Coherence Tomography

Doppler OCT is mainly used for measuring the flow of fluids within blood vessels and microvessel morphology. It works similar to Doppler acoustic imaging where the speed of moving particles alters the frequencies of backscattered light and this helps in obtaining functional images. The main alteration in this type is within the detector, which is locked at a certain frequency that indicates the depth at which light is reflected. Any alteration to this value adds to the Doppler effect [217].

12.4.1.1.5. Differential Absorption Optical Coherence Tomography

Differential absorption OCT makes use of two different wavelength light sources in the process of imaging. One will be more than the absorption peak of selected tissue, and the other will be lesser. This helps in the validation of structural and functional abnormalities for a selected tissue specimen [217].

12.4.1.1.6. Molecular Optical Coherence Tomography

Molecular OCT makes use of the differential light absorption properties of various biomarkers in a tissue sample. It is mainly useful for detecting neoplasms and tissue oxygenation properties, where there will be alterations in the biomarkers. Optical coherence elastography mainly uses elastic modulus property of tissues for imaging, which gets altered, in cases of edema, neoplasms, calcifications, and fibrosis [10, 217-219].

OCT also has been expanded for 3D imaging by adding a silicon based microelectromechanical system (MEMS) mirror to the normal 2D scanner. 3D images were obtained by combining both transverse and longitudinal scans of MEMS scanner with the axial scanning of rapid scanning optical delay [217-219].

12.4.2. Applications of Dental OCT

12.4.2.1. Oral Vascular Malformation

Ozawa et al. 2009 detected two cases of vascular malformation, one with a capillary-venous malformation of the lower lip whereas the other with a reddish mass on the buccal mucosa. In these cases, OCT images correlated well with histological structures, exhibiting well-demarcated capillary vessel lumina and endothelial lining. Cognizance of the size, area, and the border of the vascular lesions can be subsidiary for the diagnosis and cull of surgical treatment, particularly for vascular anomalies, and hemangiomas in the oromaxillofacial region [10].

12.4.2.2. Mucocutaneous Lesions

There is a certain skin disorder, which is detected by OCT. However, it requires specific attention for skin disorders whose incidence is additionally higher in the oral cavity, like lichen planus, pemphigus, pemphigoid, and so on. Forsea et al. had done studies of three patients with psoriasis and concluded that OCT showed typical thickening of the epidermis, with epidermal protrusion into the dermis, vigorous hyperkeratosis as a more tenebrous superficial band. Forsea et al. had detected sarcoidosis with OCT. There were hypo-dense confluent rounded structures in the dermis, corresponding on the histopathology exam to granulomatous infiltrates [10, 218].

Principles: [10, 217-219]

1. When OCT is used for oral cancer diagnosis, the main features to take into account are the grade of keranitization, epithelial thickening, epithelial irregular stratification, epithelial proliferation/down growth, and basal hyperplasia [30]. Since changes occur in oral cancer lesions with respect to normal tissue, an additional OCT image is taken from the healthy tissue close to the lesion for comparison.
2. In mild to severe dysplasia and CIS progression, the epithelial layer will still appear well defined and separated from the connective tissue beneath, but it is usually thicker than normal.
3. In cases of early-stage and well-developed squamous cell carcinoma (SCC), the boundaries between the epithelial layer and the lamina propria and their architecture are disrupted. This peculiar feature is extremely useful in identifying lesion borders between areas that are clearly stratified and those that are disorganized and in which layers are no longer clearly

distinguishable. Another indicator of SCC is a highly heterogeneous appearance of the epithelial layer due to the presence of cancer cell nests.

4. Malignancy is also highlighted by the presence of connective tissue papilla (CTP). Early-stage SCC (ES-SCC) is characterized by a high density of CTP, which decreases with cancer progression.
5. The evaluation of epithelial thickness could be used as an indicator of the presence of epithelial hyperplasia or moderate dysplasia. They also observed that a high standard deviation of the A-Scan along the epithelial layer highlights the heterogeneity of cell organization, giving a fingerprint for cancer cell nests. The presence of CTP and their density could be scored by looking at the standard deviation of pixel values along a line parallel to the surface at a depth of 350 μm. A high variability indicates high density, hence ES-SCC. On the other hand, a low variability suggests low CTP density and therefore a higher cancer stage. Tsai et al. also observed a higher axial light attenuation in WD-SCC, probably due to the presence of blood capillaries. For this reason, they suggested the exponential decay constant of the average A-scan intensity profile as a parameter to distinguish between well-differentiated (WD)-SCC and ES-SCC.
6. Statistical analysis of the data confirmed the capability of *in vivo* OCT for detecting and diagnosing oral premalignancy and malignancy in human subjects, with an excellent intraobserver agreement between OCT scores.

12.4.3. Limitations of Optical Coherence Tomography [217-219]

1. Contrast in OCT is mainly because of light scattering, whereas with respect to histopathology it is mainly because of specific

strains that are being used. Hence, it can be stated that OCT is not analogous to histopathological examination.
2. When there is any strong absorption or scattering of light due to haemorrhage, there will be strong attenuation of light and shadowing of deeper structures, leading to the decreased diagnostic value of the final image.
3. The depth of penetration is limited to 1.5–2 mm. Thus, definitive identification of basement membrane is difficult.
4. Most of the oral premalignancies are often associated with hyperkeratosis, which in turn has a negative influence on image quality.

12.4.4. Advantages of OCT [10, 218]

1. Non-invasive
2. High-resolution
3. Repeatability
4. Reduces the chances of further spread of infection
5. Capability to distinguish different layers like epithelial and sub-epithelial layers
6. Patient friendliness
7. Live subsurface images at a near-microscopic resolution
8. Instantaneous direct imaging of tissue morphology
9. Preparation of the sample or subject is not required
10. No contact is made with the patient
11. No use of ionizing radiation.

12.5. Confocal Laser Endomicroscopy

Confocal laser endomicroscopy (CLE) is an adaptation of white-light microscopy in which tissue and cellular structures are visualized by stimulating the emission of light using a low-power laser beam after the application of fluorescent contrast agents (Wright and Wright 2002). The image of the scanned region can be constructed and digitized by measuring the light returning to the detector. A series of confocal images can be used to observe fine cellular or sub-cellular structures, and three-dimensional structures in the specimen can also be reconstructed—thus CLE provides a tool for "optical biopsy" in the clinic (De Palma 2009). CLE holds promise for image-guided surgery by aiding in the assessment of lesion margins during surgical procedures (Nguyen et al. 2009; Pogorzelski et al. 2012). Recently, Nathan et al. (2014) conducted a prospective study of 21 patients with leukoplakia and cancerous head and neck lesions; the results showed that the diagnosis based on CLE correlated well with histopathology [220].

12.6. Photodynamic Diagnosis

Photodynamic diagnosis (PDD) is based on the fluorescence generated by the administration of an exogenous photo activated compound that accumulates in cells with malignant potential, followed by appropriate photo irradiation (Uekusa et al. 2010). One of the most promising photosensitizers for oral PMDs and oral cancer diagnosis is 5-aminolevulinic acid (ALA), which does not fluoresce itself, but can induce protoporphyrin IX (PPIX) fluorescence in the tissue. PDD in the oral cavity can be performed simply by rinsing with a 0.4% ALA solution for 20 min (Zenk et al. 1999). Topical application of excessive 5-ALA stimulates the production and intracellular accumulation of highly fluorescent PPIX in dysplastic and cancerous tissues, which is excited by brief exposure to light with a wavelength of 405 nm (Chang and Wilder-Smith 2005). Fluorescent tissues are considered suspicious for malignant transformation and biopsy should be considered (Driemel et al. 2007). A high sensitivity but limited specificity of PDD in the detection of oral PMDs and oral cancer has been shown in several studies (Leunig et al. 2000; Sharwani et al. 2006b). The false-positive rate is especially high in patients who have a history of radiotherapy (Zenk et al. 1999). Given that various bacterial strains in the oral cavity can also produce PPIX under incubation of 5-ALA (Zenk et al. 1999), professional hygiene measures must be employed before PDD in order to increase the specificity. The need for an interval of about one hour between hygiene measures and the application of photosensitizing 5-ALA, as well as about three hours between the application of 5-ALA and the formation of a sufficient level of PPIX for fluorescence measurement, limits the use of this method in outpatient cancer prevention and aftercare. Moreover, even low levels of glucose can influence PPIX production; thus, patients must fast during the four hours necessary for examination, which requires strict patient management. To improve the diagnostic specificity, a 5-ALA mediated fluorescence endoscopic imaging system has been built (Zheng et al. 2002). When PPIX fluorescence endoscopic images are quantified, the red-to-green and red-to-blue intensity ratios of dysplasia and malignancy are larger than those of benign tissues (Zheng et al. 2002; Bigio and Bown 2004). Zheng et al. (2004) quantified the red-to-blue intensity ratio in the ALA-induced PPIX fluorescence endoscopic images and showed that it could provide good differentiation between benign dysplasia and cancer. Wang et al. (2009) found that oral submucous fibrosis mucosa had the lowest red-to-blue intensity ratio, and their results indicated that ALA-induced PPIX fluorescence spectroscopy could be used to identify oral submucous fibrosis. Moreover, in a study of 71 patients with clinically suspicious oral leukoplakia, Sharwani et al. (2006b) found that ALA-induced PPIX fluorescence spectroscopy had great potential for identifying dysplastic changes at an early stage and might be useful as a screening tool for the detection of subsequent primary lesions [10, 220].

12.7. Laser Spectroscopy

RS is a vibrational spectroscopy method based on the inelastic scattering of light. Sir C. V. Raman discovered inelastic scattering of light, also known as Raman effect, after seminal experiments on scattering. When a sample is irradiated with intense monochromatic light, phenomena such as absorption, scattering, and reflection occur. Most of the scattered photons have the same frequency of the incident light (Rayleigh scattering) while a small proportion (one in ten million) are inelastically scattered, i.e., with a frequency different from the incident photons; this phenomenon is termed as Raman effect. When the frequency of the scattered light is lower than the frequency of the incident photon, the process is called Stokes shift. If the frequency of the scattered photon is higher than the incident photon, the process is called anti-stokes shift. The energy difference between the incident and scattered photon (Raman shift) is represented as wave number (/cm) [11, 221].

12.7.1. Instrumentation

RS is an inherently weak process: Only 1 in 10 million photons are Raman scattered. Thus, sophisticated instrumentation, i.e., powerful excitation source, high-throughput spectrograph, and sensitive detection systems are a prerequisite. The introduction of a low-noise charged coupled device (CCD) detector technology, highly efficient imaging spectrographs, and compact semiconductor laser excitation sources enabled extensive Raman spectroscopic applications in diverse areas.

Typically, Raman spectrometer is made up of (i) excitation source, (ii) optical system, (iii) spectrograph, and (iv) detection and computer control/processing systems. For most applications, a continuous-wave laser is employed as the excitation source in Raman spectrometers. The optical system consists of light steering mechanisms, which direct and select laser wavelength for sample excitation. Rayleigh rejection system, which prevents elastically scattered light to be incident on the spectrograph and detector, is the most crucial component of Raman system as it facilitates the rejection of Rayleigh scattered light and detection of the comparatively weaker Raman scattered light. The main function of the spectrograph is to disperse light into its component wavelengths [221].

Within biological tissues four principal components contribute to the spectra; water, lipids (cell membranes), nucleic acids (DNA and RNA), and proteins (hormones, isoenzymes, immunoglobulins, and keratins). The resultant spectra from these structures give a characteristic signature for that tissue. The operator can change the wavelength and hence can probe different depths of tissue due to different wavelength penetrations and the technique, therefore, represents a true form of optical histochemistry. The major disadvantage of this technique is that it is expensive and complex [222].

Stone N et al. (2000) used Raman spectroscopy to differentiate premalignant and malignant lesions from normal laryngeal mucosa. They concluded that there was strong evidence to support spectral identification of malignancy and earlier abnormal changes [223]. Lau et al. (2003) investigated the reliability of Raman spectroscopy in differentiating between normal and cancerous tissue. They suggested that Raman spectroscopy could be a useful tool to distinguish cancer from normal tissue [224]. Malini R et al. (2006) used Raman spectroscopy for discrimination of normal, inflammatory, premalignant, and malignant oral tissue. They concluded that the biochemical differences between normal and pathological conditions of oral tissue showed different classes of spectra, hence discriminating the lesions [225].

12.8. Laser Flowcytometry

Flow cytometry is a widespread and powerful technique employed in cell counting, biomarker detection, and cell sorting. After the Coulter Principle was discovered in 1953 and Fulwyler applied this principle to sort cells in 1965, optical detections were soon adopted by flow cytometry and fluorescence-activated cell sorter (FACS) systems since the late 1960s [226]. Soon afterward, when false positive occurrence became a concern, imaging-in-flow techniques, including flying spot scanners, slit-imaging onto an array, laser strobes, and mirror tracking, were seen as invaluable in understanding discrepancies in cell measurements due to cell orientation and dynamics in fluid flow. At the same time, because of flow cytometry's successful applications in immunology with the growing appreciation of researchers for the complexity of the immune system, further technological advances have focused on satisfying the increasing need for polychromatic approaches to flow cytometry; researchers have developed flow cytometry to simultaneously measure 19 parameters—17 fluorescence and 2 scatter parameters in a high-speed manner [227].

Flow cytometry is the process in which cells in an isotonic buffer suspension pass through a laser beam one by one. Quantifiable measurements of cellular attributes, such as cell size, granularity, DNA/RNA content, surface, and intracellular receptors, and gene expression, are made using the principle of fluorescence, or excited light energy [228]

The flow cytometer consists of four systems: fluidics, optics, electronics, and computer interface [229-231].

The first step is fluidics. Cellular suspensions, the most common source of material used in flow cytometry for disease characterization and usually derived from blood, tissue, or tumours, are labelled using fluorochrome-labelled monoclonal antibodies. Anti-bodies are proteins that recognize and bind to specific antigen structures on the cell surface, or intracellularly, to identify the measurement(s) of interest. Fluorochromes, compounds that emit light when excited, are bound to the antibodies. The fluorochrome-labelled cells in the liquid suspension then pass individually and rapidly through a laser beam sensing area.

Optics consists of the light-amplification source (laser). The laser emits light of a specified wavelength. There are several types of lasers, each capable of exciting specific fluorochromes and causing them to emit light. Once the suspension passes the laser, two initial detections are made. Forward scatter (FSC) is light that scatters in the same direction as the laser and is indicative of cellular morphology or cell size. Side scatter (SSC) is light that is scattered at a 90 degrees angle from the direction of the laser and is proportional to cell granularity (structures within the cell), or cell density.

The electronics involve the conversion of photons into interpretable data. The flow cytometer's photomultiplier tubes (PMTs) are semiconductors that generate electrical current based on light detection. The PMTs will convert the detected photons into electrical signals that can be interpreted. Each signal detected by the cytometer is known as an "event," and all events for a prepared sample are acquired by the cytometer and stored on the computer. The computer is also responsible for regulating the function of the flow cytometer. Graphic analysis of the samples can be interpreted in one-, two-, or three-dimensional images using software designed for flow cytometry data analysis.

Data analysis is often depicted in graphic formats and accompanies patient test results. It can be displayed in a variety of ways. Histograms display one measurement of interest, whereas dot plots display two parameters of interest. Many flow cytometers are capable of cell sorting. Cells or cell particles, such as lymphocytes or chromosomes, may be physically separated from the heterogeneous suspension and collected as a highly purified suspension. This process allows for the observation and analysis of a uniform population, for investigation. More clinically relevant, it allows for the selection of cells with particular features, often used to diagnose or treat a disease or condition.

12.8.1. Applications to Clinical Practice [226-232]

Flow cytometry is often used to characterize diseases in clinical settings. Peripheral blood, bone marrow aspirate, and cerebrospinal fluid are all specimens that can be analysed using flow cytometry. However, only viable cells can be analysed. If the sample does not contain viable cells, flow cytometry analysis is not an option. Flow cytometry is most commonly indicated for both benign and malignant haematologic processes.

Table 28. Summary of imaging flow cytometry (IFC) techniques [232]

Features	Image Stream	Multiple-view	Temporally coded Excitation	STEAM	FIRE	Spatial–temporal transformation
Illumination (spectral range)	LASER	LED	LASER	PULSE LASER (near infrared)	LASER	LASER
Detector	LED TDI CCD	CMOS	LED CMOS	Single Pixel Detector	PMT	PMT
Modality	Florescence Transmission Side scatter	Transmission	Florescence Transmission	Transmission Phase Contrast	Florescence	Florescence Transmission Back scatter
Data transfer & computation Complexity	Simple	Simple	Simple	Complex	Complex	Simple
Inherit functions from FC	Yes	No	Yes	No	Yes	Yes
Compatibility with sorting	No	No	No	No	No	Yes
Image resolution	Moderate	Moderate	High	Moderate	High	Moderate
Throughput (cells per s)	Upto 1,000	Approx 10,000	Approx 2,000	Upto 1,00,000	Approx 50,000	>1,000
Real-time processing solution	Yes	No	No	Yes	No	Yes

It can aid in several clinical areas, including diagnosis, treatment plans, and monitoring residual or relapsed disease. Measurement of DNA content was one of the earliest uses of flow cytometry. A 67% increase in DNA content was noted in malignant cells compared with non-malignant cells (Barlogie et al., 1983). Normal, healthy cells are diploid (two complete sets of chromosomes), whereas malignant cells most often have abnormalities in their chromosomes, which can be quantified by flow cytometry. Phenotyping, the identification of specific observable characteristics, is another common use of flow cytometry in oncology. There are many phenotypic designations to differentiate healthy cells from tumor cells. Tumour cells often express distinguishable surface receptors. For example, flow cytometry analysis of patients with acute promyelocytic leukemia (APL) has been shown to demonstrate a myeloid phenotype as CD11b$_{-}$ and CD11c$_{-}$.

In contrast, in normal myeloid cells, the phenotype is CD11b$_{+}$ and CD11c$_{+}$. The designation of T-cell or B-cell lineage in acute lymphoblastic leukemias (ALLs) is another example of phenotyping. Once denoted T-cell or B-cell ALL, each lineage can be refined by further immunoprofiling to determine subgroups and prognosis. Varma and Naseem (2011) have described the phenotype of each subgroup in detail. A pre– B-cell leukemia will express CD19 and CD10, whereas a mature B-cell leukemia will express CD19 but not CD10. Understanding the specific origin of B-cell leukemia assists in treatment options and prognosis. Several nurse-led research projects have used flow cytometry to enhance clinical understanding and to evaluate the physiologic effects of nursing interventions. It was used to evaluate the immune function of geriatric patients who received nutritional supplementation before and after flu shots. Flow cytometry has also been used to examine the immune function of caregivers of patients with Alzheimer's disease. This has been also used to examine natural killer and T-cell function in correlation to the psychological distress of patients with irritable bowel syndrome. Since women experience immunosuppression during pregnancy, flow cytometry has been used to examine the immune state of postpartum women over time.

A summary of imaging flow-cytometry techniques has been provided in Table 28.

Chapter 13

Miscellaneous Applications of Lasers

13.1. Role in Dentinal Hypersensitivity

Erbium, CO_2, Nd:YAG, and surgical diode lasers are frequently used to treat dentinal hypersensitivity. Studies mainly focus on the obliteration of the dentinal tubules but disregard the laser's additional bio stimulatory effect. LLLT will not modify the dentinal tubules but will produce an effect in the odontoblastic layer, stimulate secondary dentin formation, and simultaneously reduce inflammation. In combination with traditional desensitizing agents, LLLT is a valuable treatment modality. Ladalardo et al. studied the influence of different wavelengths on pain reduction and found the 660-nm red diode was more effective than the 830-nm IR diode laser [10, 11].

13.2. Sinusitis

Reduced breathing capacity through the nostrils is a problem for both the patient and dentist. LLLT at 3 to 4 J into the nostrils, or extraorally over the base of the nostrils, will reduce the oedema and facilitate breathing by opening the airways. The obstruction of the airways may be caused by infection or chronic allergy; sinusitis may result from dental conditions or infection. The dentist can alleviate symptoms, primarily by irradiating intraorally over the projection of the maxillary sinuses, 10 to 15 J, until the patient reports reduced pressure. The frontal and ethmoidal sinuses may be included in the irradiation therapy. The literature is scarce, and antibiotics for bacterial sinusitis are still the first choice. However, the dental session can be facilitated by adding the laser [12].

13.3. Somatosensory Tinnitus

In cases of somatosensory tinnitus, the lateral pterygoid muscles are often involved. Typically, the left muscle is tender on palpation with premature contact on the contralateral side, whereas both left and right pterygoid muscles are frequently involved with premature contact anteriorly. Premature contacts press the condyle into a retarded position, triggering a nociceptive reflex in the lateral pterygoid, trying to pull the condyle forward. A comprehensive occlusal analysis is followed by careful removal of interferences, and then the tender points in the involved muscles are irradiated to facilitate recovery. The patient should receive information about posture and stress management. Muscles as far inferiorly as the trapezius are within the dental area in temporomandibular disorders and easily treatable with the laser. Energies are chosen through patient feedback, typically 10 to 15 J per point, depending on the size of the muscle [12].

13.4. Laser Acupuncture

In dentistry, acupuncture and laser acupuncture are used in the following conditions: [11, 12]

1. Pain Control. Points ST6 ST7 L14 are considered general stimulation points for facial pain relief and the induction of analgesia during small oral surgery procedures, for temporomandibular joint disorders, or myo-fascial pain [11, 12].
2. Gag Reflex. Points PC6 (the one mostly used) and CV24 individually or in combination. This method is widely used in all those conditions where excessive oral stimulation induces an abnormal gag reflex (e.g., during the taking of casts or to perform intraoral radiographs) or for vomiting induced by anticancer drugs or in the vomiting after surgery, without any adverse effect compared with antiemetic drugs [11, 12].
3. Hyposalivation. A reduction in saliva flow determined by pathological conditions of the salivary glands, or as a side effect of radio- and chemotherapy, or by physiological glandular involution, generates a progressive deterioration of oral health. In scientific literature, there are studies that have used the stimulation of acupuncture points to increase the salivary flow, obtaining persistent good results. In addition to points located on the face (ST6 ST7 ST5 SI19), points are used in other parts of the body (limbs and trunk) in relation to the energy imbalance of the subjects enrolled in the various studies [11, 12].
4. Anxiety Control. Many patients live with extreme anxiety in dental sessions; the stimulation of acupuncture points on the ear allows greater control of the levels of anxiety and stress. The wavelengths used in laser acupuncture are 400 nm (blue), 635 nm (red) which is the most common, 700– 1000 nm (infrared) which has a greater depth of penetration, and 532 nm (green) mainly used for the auriculotherapy, but few studies can be found in the literature. Regarding the dose to be administered as well as the repetition of treatments, there are no guidelines, a dose range, in accordance with Litscher G. and Opitz G. between 0.001 and 10 J/cm^2, and therapy sessions every other day for diseases in the acute stage and once a week for chronic conditions are generally considered correct [11, 12].

13.5. ANTIMICROBIAL PHOTODYNAMIC THERAPY [10-12]

Antimicrobial photodynamic therapy (aPDT), also known as photodynamic inactivation (PDI) [10-12], photo activated disinfection (PAD) or photodynamic antimicrobial chemotherapy (PACT), is a non-invasive method, an alternative or an adjunctive treatment to chemical agents in order to eliminate the bacteria in oral infections such as periodontitis and peri-implantitis.

1. Periodontitis. A significant reduction of *Aggregatibacter actinomycetemcomitans*, *Porphyromonas gingivalis*, and *Prevotella intermedia* after treatment with TBO-mediated PDT has been reported. In vitro using poly (lactic-co-glycolic) (PLGA) nanoparticles as carriers of MB. The results suggested that PLGA nanoparticles have the potential to be used as nanocarriers of MB, to increase diffusion into biofilms, and to help release the encapsulated drug in active form. They showed a greater PDT bacterial killing.
2. Endodontic disinfection. Garcez et al. used PDT to kill Gram-negative (*Pseudomonas aeruginosa* and *Proteus mirabilis*) bacteria growing as biofilms in root canals of extracted teeth.
3. Viral lesions. Clinical studies on infectious diseases have tested PDT to treat herpes simplex lesions. Herpes keratitis was healed by proflavine photodynamic viral inactivation. In other studies, photo inactivation of herpes virus with neutral red was found to be ineffective.
4. Oral candidiasis. The effectiveness of PDT has also been evaluated in the inactivation of *C. albicans* in oral candidiasis. Recently, Mima et al. evaluated the efficacy of using hematoporphyrin with PDT in an animal model of oral candidiasis. In this study, candidiasis was verified by the presence of white patches or pseudomembranes on the dorsal

tongue associated with a significant number of colony-forming units (CFU)/mL of *C. albicans*, and PDT significantly reduced the viability of *C. albicans*.

5. PDT in caries. The change in emphasis towards minimally invasive procedures in modern dentistry places antimicrobial PDT in a promising position. The ability of PDT mediated by phenothiazinum dyes (commonly TBO and MB) to efficiently kill bacteria in cariogenic biofilms existing on enamel surfaces and in infected dentin structures, even if located in hard to reach regions such as bifurcations and fissures, turns this technique into a unique tool. Furthermore, the possibility of enabling the remineralization of affected tissues through a biological or therapeutic approach is currently a promising strategy in dentistry, reducing drastically the invasiveness of traditional restorative treatments.

13.6. Lasers in Caries Prevention [10, 12]

1. CO_2 laser irradiation combined with topical fluoride treatment can induce an even greater increase in caries resistance. There are two possible mechanisms for the laser-induced increase of fluoride uptake. In the first mechanism, the laser–fluoride treatment produces numerous spherical precipitates, that morphologically resemble calcium fluoride-like deposits on the dental surfaces, which serve as a reservoir to replenish fluoride. However, no calcium fluoride formation is seen on the enamel surface when the CO_2 laser is used alone. The second mechanism emphasizes the role of lasers in enhancing fluoride uptake into the crystalline structure of the tooth in the form of firmly bound fluoride.
2. The proposed mechanism for the protective effect of argon laser irradiation against both caries initiation and progression is the alteration of the characteristics of the enamel surface by creating

micro spaces that trap calcium, phosphate, and fluoride ions during an acid challenge. The ions are incorporated into the enamel surface. In other words, in the lased enamel, the micro spaces trap the released ions and act as sites for mineral reprecipitation within the enamel structure. Thus, the enamel irradiated with the argon laser has an increased affinity for calcium, phosphate, and fluoride ions.

3. As studies have reported surface melting and temperatures of up to 600°C when the enamel is irradiated with Nd:YAG lasers, similar mechanisms to those for CO_2 lasers have been suggested for Nd:YAG lasers in caries prevention. However, unlike the CO_2 laser, which is the most efficiently absorbed laser by dental enamel, the Nd:YAG laser is not effectively absorbed by human enamel (the absorption coefficient is lower than 4 × 101–2/cm) [21]. Thus, its efficient use in this substrate depends on the application of a photosensitizer.

13.7. Laser Induced Tooth Analgesia

The Er,Cr:YSGG (2780 nm) laser can be used by applying a combination between *rabbit* and modified *turtle techniques*. The study of laser-induced dental analgesia with regard to cavity preparation was performed by adopting the following sequence: [11, 12].

1. A preliminary pulp test using the electric pulp tester to evaluate dental vitality and to establish the baseline threshold of dental sensitivity.
2. Beginning of the dental analgesia induction phase by using power settings of 0.1 and then 0.2 W (energy per pulse of 10 and 20 mJ) at a pulse repetition rate of 10 Hz, for 30 s each (without using any air/water cooling spray), keeping the tip at 10 mm from the tooth using a spacer. Subsequently, the power was increased to 0.5 and then to 1 W (energy per pulse of 33 and 67

mJ) for 60 s each, with a spray composed by 15% of water (for our laser this means approximately 10 ml/min) and 20% of air, at a pulse repetition rate of 15 Hz, keeping the tip at the same distance from the tooth neck.

3. Preconditioning of hard tissues with 2 W of power for 30 s with a cooling spray of 50% water (approximately 20 ml/min) and 80% air, at 15 Hz of pulse repetition rate, with the tip at approximately 1 mm from the tooth. The laser beam was kept in focus or, if the patient felt discomfort, it was defocused according to sensitivity.
4. Electric pulp test (EPT) performed again to evaluate the presence of analgesia and establish how the threshold value of dental sensitivity had changed. Preconditioning and beginning of enamel ablation with a 3 W power for 30 s (same previous settings as for pulse repetition rate, distance, and cooling spray).

13.8. Lasers in Sterilization

Micro-organisms induce a variety of infectious diseases in the human body. Infection control is a major topic of concern in medical and dental health care settings. Contamination directly or indirectly leads to the transmission of infectious agents. The prevention of cross-contamination of infectious diseases among dental staff and patients is a major problem, which dental practitioners face. Sterilization prevents the spread of infectious diseases. In dentistry, it primarily relates to processing reusable instruments to prevent cross-infection. CO_2 laser technology is being used as one of the modes of sterilization nowadays in the dental office. CO_2 laser used for sterilization shows complete sterilization of the endodontic instruments as presented by Nammour et al. Powell et al. on the basis of a study stated that all 3 lasers (argon, CO_2, and NdYAG) were capable of sterilizing endodontic instruments, but the efficiency of argon laser was better even at lower energy level [226].

13.9. USE OF LASERS IN OTHER FIELDS OF DENTISTRY

Lasers are called the miracle device, which can be implemented, in all fields of dentistry. In Orthodontics, LLLT can be used for reduction of post-activation and post-adjustment pain, bone regeneration in mid-palatine suture after rapid maxillary expansion, and acceleration of tooth movement. In the speciality of Preventive, aesthetic, and restorative dentistry, lasers can be employed for selective caries removal, aesthetic, improvement in adhesion to dental tissues, management of non-carious cervical lesions, dental bleaching, treatment of internal ceramic surfaces, etc. Lasers can be used for antimicrobial PDT of the root canal system and apical surgery. Lasers also can be used as a minimally invasive procedure to improve outcomes in fields of Implantology, Bone biomodulation, Pre-prosthetic surgeries, and Obstructive sleep apnoea [10, 11, 12].

CONCLUSION

"To know is to use. To understand is to empower…" [11]

Lasers have been suggested as an alternative or adjunctive to conventional techniques for various dental procedures and considered superior with respect to easy ablation, decontamination, and haemostasis along with less operative and post-operative pain. Given its incredibly diverse use on soft tissue and its versatility, it can be regarded as a "Soft-tissue Handpiece" in a dentist's armamentarium. Although the range of conditions able to be treated is wide, it requires some technical expertise and knowledge, but for most doctors, physiotherapists, and allied health professionals, the learning curve is small, and a judicious practitioner can well incorporate this technology in day-to-day practice. Successful outcomes, like all medical management, depend on integrating individual clinical expertise with the best available external clinical evidence from systematic research.

Biophotonics in Dentistry, with its ramifications into photo diagnosis, photo detection, and phototherapeutics is crucial for the early detection of diseases, to carry out more effective minimally invasive targeted therapies and to restore diseased tissues functionally and aesthetically. Biophotonics offers a remarkable prospectus for both clinical applications and fundamental research. In the future, biophotonics is anticipated to play a major role in creating new technologies for significant health care benefits and immense commercial potential for different biomedical industries. Future opportunities with biophotonics are development and testing of multiple-analyte-based nano-probes, optical biosensors for infections and cancers, in vivo optical biopsy, tissue welding, tissue contouring, and regeneration, in vivo imaging of human subjects, real-time monitoring of drug delivery and action. All these technological aids should be supported by long-term clinical evaluations [4]

REFERENCES

[1] May HG. The Creation of Light in Genesis 1:3-5. *Journal of Biblical Literature* 1939 Sep; 58(3):203-211.

[2] Ott JN. *Health and Light: The Effects of Natural and Artificial Light on Man and Other Living Things*. London: Ariel Press; 1973.

[3] Al-Amri MD, El-Gomati MM, Zubairy MS, editors. *Optics in Our Time*. Switzerland: Springer Nature; 2016.

[4] Kishen A, Asundi A. *Fundamentals and Applications of Biophotonics in Dentistry*. London: Imperial College Press; 2007.

[5] Gujjar KR, Sumra N. Minimally Invasive Dentistry - A Review. *International Journal of Clinical Preventive Dentistry* 2013 June; 9(2):109-120.

[6] Prasad PN. *Introduction to Biophotonics*. New Jersey: Wiley Interscience Inc.; 2003.

[7] Maiman comments on his precocious five-year old (editorial), *Laser Focus* 1(9):2-4, 1965.

[8] Verma SK, Maheshwari S, Singh RK, Chaudhari PK. Laser in dentistry: An innovative tool in modern dental practice. *Natl J Maxillofac Surg*. 2012 Jul-Dec; 3(2): 124–132.

[9] Walsh LJ. The current status of laser applications in dentistry. *Aust Dent J*. 2003; 48:146–55.

[10] de Freitas PM, Simões A, editors. *Lasers in Dentistry Guide for Clinical Practice*. 1st ed. Wiley Blackwell; 2015.

[11] Coluzzi DJ, Parker SPA, editors. *Lasers in Dentistry—Current Concepts*. Switzerland: Springer Nature; 2017.

[12] Convissar RA. 2nd ed. *Principles and Practice of Laser Dentistry*. China: Mosby Elsevier; 2016.

[13] Gribbin JR: Q is for quantum: an encyclopedia of particle physics, New York, 2000, Touchstone.

[14] Opera omnia ... haetenus edita auctor ante obitum recensuit... posthuma vero, totius naturae explicationen complectentia, in lucem nunc primum proderunt ex bibliotheca ... Henrici-Ludovici-Haberti Mon-Morii ... [Accesit Samuelis Sorberii praefatio, in qua de vita et moribus Petri Gassendi disseritur], Lyon, 1658, Laurent Anisson and Jean Baptiste Devenet, I, pp 422a-432b.

[15] *Newton I: Opticks: or, a treatise of the reflexions, refractions, inflexions and colours of light.* Also two treatises of the species and magnitude of curvilinear figures, London, 1704, Smith and Walford, printers to the Royal Society.

[16] Hooke R: *Micrographia; or, some physiological descriptions of minute bodies made by magnifying glasses with observations and inquiries thereupon*, London, 1665, Martyn & Allestry.

[17] Planck M: Zur theorie des gesetzes der energieverteilung im normalspektrum, *Verh Dtsch Phys Ges* 2:237-245, 1900. [On the theory of the law of energy distribution in the normal spectrum]

[18] Rutherford E: The scattering of α and β particles by matter and the structure of the atom, *Philos Mag, Series* 6, 21:669-688, 1911.

[19] Einstein A: Zur quantentheorie der strahlung [On the quantum theory of radiation], Mitt Phys Ges Zurich 18:47-62, 1916.

[20] Hecht J: *Beam: the race to make the laser*, New York, 2005, Oxford University Press.

[21] *Laser pioneer interviews* (with an introduction to laser history by Jeff Hecht), Torrance, Calif, 1985, High Tech Publications.

[22] Bromberg JL: Amazing light, *Invention & Technology Magazine* 7(4): [~8 pp], 1992 [serial on Internet]. http://www.americanheritage.com/articles/magazine/it/1992/4/1992_4_18.shtml. Accessed January 2009.

[23] Paghdiwala AF. Application of the erbium:YAG laser on hard dental tissues: measurement of the temperature changes and depths of cut. In Profio AE, editor: *Laser research in medicine, dentistry and surgery*, vol 64, ICALEO; 1988, Santa Clara, Calif, Proceedings, Toledo, Ohio, 1988, Laser Institute of America, 192-201.

[24] Goldman L: Dental applications of the laser. In Goldman L: *Biomedical aspects of the laser: the introduction of laser applications into biology and medicine*, New York, 1967, Springer-Verlag.

[25] Franck P, Henderson PW, Rothaus KO. Basics of Lasers, History, Physics, and Clinical Applications. *Clin Plastic Surg* 2016; 43:505–513.

[26] Mishra MB, Mishra S. Lasers and its clinical applications in dentistry. *International Journal of Dental Clinics* 2011; 3(4): 35-38.

[27] Dyer PE, Snelling HV. Gas lasers for medical applications. Helena Jelínková, editor. *Lasers for Medical Applications-Diagnostics, Therapy and Surgery*. Woodhead publishing; 2013: p. 177-202.

[28] Šulc J, Jelínková, H. Solid state lasers for medical applications. Helena Jelínková, editor. *Lasers for Medical Applications-Diagnostics, Therapy and Surgery*. Woodhead publishing; 2013: p. 127-176.

[29] Haley D, Pratt O, *Basic principles of lasers, Anaesthesia and intensive care medicine* (2017), https://doi.org/10.1016/j.mpaic.2017.10.001.

[30] Dahiya A, Rana M, Hooda A, Arora T, Kumar A. Laser Physics: Recent Clinical Trends. *International Journal of Laser Dentistry,* September-December 2014;4(3):74-78.

[31] Fuller TA, editor. *Surgical laser: a clinical guide*. Macmillan; 1987. p. 45-50.

[32] Dederich DN. *Laser tissue interaction*. Alpha Omegan 1991;84(4):33-36.

[33] Dederick DN. Laser/tissue interaction: what happens to laser light when it strikes tissue? *JADA* 1993;124:57-61.

[34] Anderson R, Parrish J. Selective photothermolysis: precise microsurgery by selective absorption of pulsed radiation. *Science* 1983;220(4596):524–7.

[35] Kumar B, Kashyap N, Avinash A, Munot H, Pawar P, Das P. The hazardous effects and safety measures of lasers in dentistry: A review. *International Journal of Contemporary Dental and Medical Reviews* 2017; 1-5.

[36] Singh S, Gambhir RS, Singh AKG, Sharma S, Heena Kakar. Dental Lasers: A Review of Safety Essentials. *Journal of Lasers in Medical Sciences* 2012; 3(3):91-96.

[37] Coluzzi DJ. Fundamentals of dental lasers: Science and instruments. *Dent Clin North Am* 2004;48:751-70.

[38] Navratil L, Kymplova J. Contraindications in Noninvasive Laser Therapy: Truth and Fiction. *Journal of Clinical Laser Medicine & Surgery* 2002; 20(6): 341–343.

[39] Shields TD, O'Kane S, Gilmore WS. (1992). The effect of laser irradiation upon human mononuclear leukocytes. *Lasers Surg. Med. Suppl.* 4, 11.

[40] Pöntinen, PJ. (1992). *Low-Level Laser Therapy as a Medical Treatment Modality*. Tampere: Art Urpo.

[41] Cheetham M, Young S, Dyson M. (1991). 820-nm irradiation of the healthy growth plate. *Lasers Surg. Med. Suppl.* 3, 12.

[42] Navrátil L. et al. (1999). *Noninvasive Laser Therapy*. Praha: Manus.

[43] Martin DM, Baxter GD, Allen JM. (1991). Effect of laser pulse repetition rate upon peripheral blood flow in human volunteers. *Lasers Surg. Med. Suppl.* 3, 83.

[44] Rochkind S, Vogler I, Barr-Nea L. (1990). Spinal cord response to laser treatment of injured peripheral nerve. *Spine* 15, 6–10. 22. Hasan, P.

[45] Piccione PJ. Dental laser safety. *Dent Clin North Am* 2004;48:795-807.

[46] Leo M, Robert P, Blankenau R. *Laser safety in dental practice. Lasers in Dentistry*. Chicago: Quintessence Publishing; 1995. p. 85-99.

[47] Goyal M, Makkar S, Pasricha S. Low Level Laser Therapy in Dentistry. *International Journal of Laser Dentistry*, September-December 2013;3(3):82-88.

[48] Grace Sun, Jan Tuner. Low-level laser therapy in dentistry. *Dent Clin N Am* 48 (2004); 1061–1076.

[49] Mester E, Spiry T, Szende B, et al. Effect of laser-rays on wound healing. *Am J Surg* 1971; 22:532–5.

[50] Saquib S, Jadhav V, Priyanka N, Perla N. Low-level laser therapy in dentistry: A review. *International Journal of Contemporary Dental and Medical Reviews* 2014; 1-3.

[51] Kathuria V, Dhillon JK, Kalra G. Low Level Laser Therapy: A Panacea for oral maladies. *Laser Therapy* 24.3: 215-223.

[52] Huang YY, Chen CHA. Biphasic dose response in low level light therapy. *Formerly Nonlinearity in Biology, Toxicology, and Medicine-Dose-Response* 2009; 7:358–383.

[53] Hamblin MR, Demidova TN. Mechanisms of Low Level Light Therapy. *Proceedings of SPIE - The International Society for Optical Engineering* 2006 March; 6140: 1-12.

[54] Farivar S, Malekshahabi T, Shiari R. Biological Effects of LLLT. *Journal of Lasers in Medical Sciences* 2014; 5(2): 58-62.

[55] Beltran B, Mathur A, Duchen MR, Erusalimsky JD, Moncada S. The effect of nitric oxide on cell respiration: A key to understanding its role in cell survival or death, *Proc Natl Acad Sci USA* 2000; 97(26):14602-7.

[56] Karu T. Primary and secondary mechanisms of action of visible to near-IR radiation on cells. *J Photochem Photobiol* 1999; 49(1):1-17.

[57] Walsh LJ. The current status of low level laser therapy in dentistry. Part 1. Soft tissue applications. *Australian Dental Journal* 1997;42:(4):247-54.

[58] de Morais NC, Barbosa AM, Vale ML et al. Anti-Inflammatory Effect of Low-Level Laser and Light-Emitting Diode in Zymosan-Induced Arthritis. *Photomed Laser Surg* 2010; 28: 227–232.

[59] Mezawa S, Iwata K, Naito K, Kamogawa H. The possible analgesic effect of soft-laser irradiation on heat nociceptors in the cat tongue. *Arch Oral Biol* 1988;33:693-4.

[60] Armida MMT. Laser therapy and its applications in dentistry. *Pract Odontol* 1989;10:9-16.

[61] Peres F, Felino A, Carvalho JF. Analgesic effect of 904-nm laser radiation (IR) in oral surgery. *Rev Port Estomatol Cir Maxilofac* 1985;26:205-17.

[62] Raab, O. *Z. Biol.,* 524 (1900). (in German).

[63] Ledoux, L. *Ann. Inst. Pasteur*, 587 (1902). (in French).

[64] Von Tappeiner H, Jodlbauer AU, *Deutsches Arch. Klin. Med.,* All (1904). (in German).

[65] Lipson RL, Baldes EJ, *Arch. Dermatol* 1960; 508.

[66] Dougherty TJ, Henderson BW, Schwartz S, Winkelman JW, Lipson RL, in *photodynamic Therapy*, Eds., BW. Henderson and TJ. Dougherty (Maurice Dekker, New York, 1992), p:1.

[67] Lustig RA, Vogl TJ, Fromm D, Cuenca R, His AR, D'Cruz AK et.al. *Cancer* 2003; 1767.

[68] Chen J, Keltner L, Christophersen J, Zheng F, Krouse M, Singhal A, Wang SS. *Cancer* 1 2003; 154.

[69] Phillips D. *Sci. Progress* 1994; 295.

[70] Foote CS, Shook FC, Abakerli RB. *Methods Enzymol* 1984; 36.

[71] Song YZ, An J, Jiang L. *Biochim. Biophys. Acta* 1999; 307.

[72] Kessel D, Luo Y, Deng Y, Chang CK. *Photochem. Photobiol* 1997; All.

[73] Wilson BC, Olivo M, Singh G. *Photochem. Photobiol* 1997; 166.

[74] Star WM, Marijnissen JP, van den Berg-Blok AE, Reinhold HS. *Prog. Clin. Biol. Res*. 1984; 637.

[75] Huang Z, Chen Q, Luck D, Beckers J, Wilson BC, Trncic N, LaRue SM, Blanc D, Hetzel FW. *Lasers Surg. Med.* 2005; 390.

[76] Nowis D, Stoklosa T, Legat M, Issat T, Jakobisiak M, Golab J. Photodiag. *Photodyn. Therapy* 2005; 283.

[77] Gollnick SO, Evans SS, Baumann H, Owczarczak B, Maier P, Vaughan L, Wang WC, Unger E, Henderson BW. *Br. J. Cancer* 2003; 1772.

[78] Korbelik M, Sun J, Cecic I, Serrano K. *Photochem Photobiol Sci.* 2004; 812.

[79] Gollnick SO, Vaughan L, Henderson BW. *Cancer Res*. 2002; 1604.

[80] Chen WR, Korbelik M, Bartels KE, Liu H, Sun J, Nordquist RE. *Photochem. Photobiol* 2005;190.

[81] Yilmaz HG, Albaba MR, Caygur A, Cengiz E, Boke-Karacaoglu F, Tumer H. Treatment of recurrent aphthous stomatitis with Er,Cr:YSGG laser irradiation: A randomized controlled split mouth clinical study. *Journal of Photochemistry & Photobiology, B: Biology* 170 (2017) 1–5.

[82] Preeti L, Magesh K, Rajkumar K, Karthik R. Recurrent aphthous stomatitis. *J Oral Maxillofac Pathol* 2011; 15(3): 252–256.

[83] James J, Burks W. Food allergies. In: Grammer LC, Greenberger PA, eds. *Pattersons's Allergic Diseases*. 7th edn. Philadelphia: Lippincott Williams & Wilkins, 2009: 315–332.

[84] Akerzoul N, Chbicheb S. Low laser therapy as an effective treatment of recurrent aphtous ulcers: a clinical case reporting two locations. *Pan African Medical Journal* 2018 Oct 7; 1-8.

[85] Jean-Paul R, Meng Z, Carlo F, Lixin T, Zengyi Z, Elisabetta M. Effect of laser irradiation on aphthae pain management: a four different wavelengths comparison. *Journal of Photochemistry & Photobiology, B: Biology* 2018.

[86] Vale FA, Moreira MS, Souza de Almeida FC, Ramalho KM. Low-Level Laser Therapy in the Treatment of Recurrent Aphthous Ulcers: A Systematic Review. *The Scientific World Journal* 2014 Oct 31; 1-7.

[87] Albrektson M, Hedström L, Bergh H. *Recurrent aphthous stomatitis and pain management with low-level laser therapy: a randomized controlled trial.* OOOO 2014 May 5; 117(5):590-594.

[88] Zand N, Fateh M, Ataie-Fashtami L, Djavid GE, Fatemi SM, Shirkavand A. Promoting Wound Healing in Minor Recurrent Aphthous Stomatitis By Non-Thermal, Non Ablative CO_2 Laser Therapy: A Pilot Study. *Photomedicine and Laser Surgery* 2012; 30(12):719-723.

[89] Pezelj-Ribarić S , Kqiku L, Brumini G, Muhvić Urek M, Antonić R, Kuiš D et al. Proinflammatory cytokine levels in saliva in patients with burning mouth syndrome before and after treatment with low-level laser therapy. *Lasers Med Sci* 2013; 28:297–301.

[90] Spanemberg JC, Segura-Egea JJ, Rivera-Campillo ER, Jané-Salas E, Salum FG, López-López J. Low-level laser therapy in patients with Burning Mouth Syndrome: A double-blind, randomized, controlled clinical trial. *J Clin Exp Dent*. 2019;11(2):162-169.

[91] Sikora M, Včev A, Siber S, Vučićević Boras V, Rotim Z, Matijević M. The efficacy of low-level laser therapy in burning mouth syndrome – a pilot study. *Acta Clin Croat* 2018; 57:312-315.

[92] Al-Maweri SA, Kalakonda FJB, Nader A. Ameen Al-Akwa AWAS. Efficacy of Low Level Laser Therapy in the Treatment of Burning Mouth Syndrome: A Systematic Review. *Photodiagnosis and Photodynamic Therapy* 2016.

[93] Sugaya NN, Patrício da SILVA EF, Kato IT, Prates R, de Barros Gallo C, Pellegrini VD. Low Intensity laser therapy in patients with burning mouth syndrome: a randomized, placebo-controlled study. *Braz. Oral Res*. 2016;30(1):1-9.

[94] dos Santos LFC, de Andrade SC, Nogueira GEC, Leao JC, de Freitas PM. Phototherapy on the Treatment of Burning Mouth

Syndrome: A Prospective Analysis of 20 Cases. *Photochemistry and Photobiology*, 2015; 91: 1231–1236.

[95] Herpich CM, Leal-Junior EC, Amaral AP, Tosato JP, Glória IPS, GarciaMBS et al. Effects Of phototherapy on muscle activity and pain in individuals with temporomandibular disorder: a study protocol for a randomized controlled trial. *Trials* 2014; 15(491): 1–8.

[96] Gonçalves DA, Dal Fabbro AL, Campos JA, Bigal ME, Speciali JG. Symptoms of temporomandibular disorders in the population: an epidemiological study. *J Orofac Pain* 2010 ; 24(3):270–278.

[97] Fbrochado FT, de Jesus LH, Carrard VC, Freddo AL, Chaves KD, Martins MD. Comparative effectiveness of photobiomodulation and manual therapy alone or combined in TMD patients: a randomized clinical trial. *Braz. Oral Res*. 2018;32(50).

[98] Xu GZ, Jia J, Jin L, Li JH, Zhan, Wang ZY, Cao DY. *Pain Research and Management* 2018.

[99] Borges RMM, Cardoso DS, Flores BC, da Luz RD, Machado CR, Cerveira GP et.al. Effects of different photobiomodulation dosimetries on temporomandibular dysfunction: a randomized, double-blind, placebo-controlled clinical trial. *Lasers in Medical Science* 2018.

[100] Demirkol N, Usumez A, Demirkol M, Sari F, Akcaboy C. Efficacy of Low-Level Laser Therapy in Subjective Tinnitus Patients with Temporomandibular Disorders. *Photomedicine and Laser Surgery* 2017; XX(XX): 1-5.

[101] Braga Cavalcanti MFX, Silva UH, Pinto Leal-Junior EC, Lopes-Martins RAB, Marcos RL, Pallotta RC et al. Comparative Study of the Physiotherapeutic and Drug Protocol and Low-Level Laser Irradiation in the Treatment of Pain Associated With Temporomandibular Dysfunction. *Photomedicine and Laser Surgery* 2016; XX(XX): 1-5.

[102] Ayyildiz S, Emir F, Sahin C. Evaluation of Low-Level Laser Therapy in TMD Patients. *Hindawi Case Reports in Dentistry* 2015.

[103] Sayed N, Murugavel C, Gnanam A. Management of Temporomandibular Disorders with Low Level Laser Therapy. *J. Maxillofac. Oral Surg* 2013.

[104] Tenis CA, Martins MD, Gonçalves MLL, Teixeira da Silva DF, Filho JJC, Trevizani Martins MA et al. Efficacy of diode-emitting diode (LED) photobiomodulation in pain management, facial edema, trismus, and quality of life after extraction of retained lower third molars-A randomized, double-blind, placebo-controlled clinical trial. Tenis et al. *Medicine* 2018; 97:37.

[105] Lauriti L, de Cerqueira Luz JG, Mesquita-Ferrari RA, Santos Fernandes KP, Deana AM, Tempestini Horliana ACR et al. Evaluation of the Effect of Phototherapy in Patients with Mandibular Fracture on Mandibular Dynamics, Pain, Edema, and Bite Force: A Pilot Study. *Photomedicine and Laser Surgery* 2017; XX(XX):1–7.

[106] Ezzat AEM, Hanna M, Shenawy EL, El-Begermy MM, Eid MI, Akel MM et.al. The effectiveness of low-level laser on postoperative pain and edema in secondary palatal operation. *International Journal of Pediatric Otorhinolaryngology* xxx (2016) 1e4.

[107] Eroglu CN, Tunc SK. Effectiveness of Single Session of Low-Level Laser Therapy with a 940nm Wavelength Diode Laser on Pain, Swelling, and Trismus After Impacted Third Molar Surgery. *Photomedicine and Laser Surgery* 2016; 34(9): 1-5.

[108] Reinheimer C, Doerr HW. Prevalence of herpes simplex virus type 2 in different risk groups: Thirty years after the onset of HIV. *Intervirology* 2012; 55(6): 395–400.

[109] Cernik C, Gallina K, Brodell RT. The treatment of herpes simplex infections: an evidence-based review. *Arch Intern Med* 2008; 168:1137–1144.

[110] Whitley RJ, Roizman B. Herpes simplex virus infections. *Lancet* 2001; 357: 1513–1518.

[111] Marotti J, Sperandio FF, Fregnani ER, Aranha AC, de Freitas PM, Eduardo Cde P. High-intensity laser and photodynamic therapy as

a treatment for recurrent herpes labialis. *Photomed Laser Surg.* 2010 Jun;28(3):439-44.

[112] Marotti J, Aranha AC, Eduardo Cde P, Ribeiro MS. Photodynamic therapy can be effective as a treatment for herpes simplex labialis. *Photomed Laser Surg.* 2009 Apr;27(2):357-63.

[113] Bello-Silva MS, de Freitas PM, Aranha AC, Lage-Marques JL, Simões A, de Paula Eduardo C. Low- and high-intensity lasers in the treatment of herpes simplex virus 1 infection. *Photomed Laser Surg.* 2010 Feb;28(1):135-9.

[114] Eduardo Cde P, Bezinelli LM, Eduardo Fde P, da Graça Lopes RM, Ramalho KM, Bello-Silva MS et al. Prevention of recurrent herpes labialis outbreaks through low-intensity laser therapy: a clinical protocol with 3-year follow-up. *Lasers Med Sci.* 2012 Sep;27(5):1077-83.

[115] de Carvalho RR, de Paula Eduardo F, Ramalho KM, Antunes JL, Bezinelli LM, de Magalhães MH et.al. Effect of laser phototherapy on recurring herpes labialis prevention: an *in vivo* study. *Lasers Med Sci.* 2010 May;25(3):397-402.

[116] Stona P, da Silva Viana E, Weber LB, Kramer PF. Recurrent Labial Herpes Simplex in Pediatric Dentistry: Low-level Laser Therapy as a Treatment Option. *International Journal of Clinical Pediatric Dentistry*, May-August 2014;7(2):140-143.

[117] Alexander B. Alveolar Osteitis: A Review of Current Concepts and Management protocols. *Journal of Dental and Medical Sciences*. September. 2018; 17(9):7-10.

[118] Ozen T, Orhan K, Gorur I, Ozturk A. Efficacy of low level laser therapy on neurosensory recovery after injury to the inferior alveolar nerve. *Head & Face Medicine* 2006, 2:3.

[119] Alayat MSM, Elsodany AM, Raouf El Fiky AA. Efficacy of high and low level laser therapy in the treatment of Bell's palsy: A randomized double blind placebo controlled trial. *Lasers Med Sci* 2013.

[120] Vernon LF. Low-level lasert for trigeminal neuralgia. *Practica Pain Management* 2008:56-63.

[121] Walker J. Relief from chronic pain by low power laser irradiation. *Neurosci Lett* 1983;43:339-44.

[122] Iijima K, Shimoyama N, Shimoyama M, Mizuguchi T. Evaluation of analgesic effect of low-power He:Ne laser on post herpetic neuralgia using VAS and modified McGill pain questionnaire. *J Clin Laser Med Surg* 1991;9:121-6.

[123] Mann SS, Dewan SP, Kaur A, Kumar P, Dhawan AK. Role of laser therapy in post herpetic neuralgia. *Indian J Dermatol Venereol Leprol* 1999;65:134-6.

[124] Moore K C, Hira N, Kramer PS, Jayakumar CS, Ohshiro T. Double blind crossover trial of low level laser therapy. *Practica Pain Management* 1988;1-7.

[125] Zand N, Mansouri P, Fateh M, Ataie-Fashtami L, Khiabanloo SR, Safar F, Chalangari R, Martits K et al. Relieving Pain in Oral Lesions of Pemphigus Vulgaris Using the Non-ablative, Non-thermal, CO_2 Laser Therapy (NTCLT): Preliminary Results of a Novel Approach. *J Lasers Med Sci* 2017 Winter;8(1):7-12.

[126] Simoes A, de Freitas PM, Bello–Silva MS, Tune J, de Paula Eduardo C. Laser Phototherapy for Stevens–Johnson Syndrome: A Case Report. *Photomedicine and Laser Surgery* 2011 Nov 1; 29(1), 2011: 67–69.

[127] Rocha AL, De Souza AF, Mendes Nunes LF, de Souza Cunha ND, Moreira Lanza CR et al. Treatment of oral manifestations of toxic epidermal necrolysis with low - level laser therapy in a pediatric patient. *Pediatric Dermatology*. 2018;1–4.

[128] Lalla RV, Bowen J, Barasch A, Elting L, Epstein J, Keefe DM, et al. Mucositis Guidelines Leadership Group of the Multinational Association of Supportive Care in Cancer and International Society of Oral Oncology (MASCC/ISOO). MASCC/ISOO clinical practice guidelines for the management of mucositis secondary to cancer therapy. *Cancer.* 2014 May 15;120(10):1453-61.

[129] Migliorati C, Hewson I, Lalla RV, Antunes HS, Estilo CL, Hodgson B et al. Systematic review of laser and other light therapy

for the management of oral mucositis in cancer patients. *Support Care Cancer*. 2013 Jan;21(1):333-41.

[130] Zecha JA, Raber-Durlacher JE, Nair RG, Epstein JB, Elad S, Hamblin MR et al. Low-level laser therapy/photobiomodulation in the management of side effects of chemoradiation therapy in head and neck cancer: part 2: proposed applications and treatment protocols. *Support Care Cancer*. 2016 Jun;24(6):2793-805.

[131] Latifyan S, Genot MT, Klastersky J. Bisphosphonate-related osteonecrosis of the jaw: a review of the potential efficacy of low-level laser therapy. *Support Care Cancer*. 2016; 24:3687–93.

[132] Paul M. Speight, Syed Ali Khurram, Omar Kujan. *Oral potentially malignant disorders: risk of progression to malignancy* 2018 June; 25(6):612-627.

[133] Yanduri S, Pandey G, Kumar VB, Suma S, Madhura MG. Artifacts in Oral Biopsy Specimens: A Comparison of Scalpel, Punch, and Laser Biopsies. *Indian Journal of Oral Health and Research* Jul-Dec 2016; 2(2):100-105.

[134] Bhatsange A, Meshram EP, Waghamare A, Shiggaon L, Mehetre V, Shende A. A clinical and histological comparison of mucosal incisions produced by scalpel, electrocautery, and diode laser: A pilot study. *Journal of Dental Lasers* July - December 2016; 2(10):37-42.

[135] Romeo U, Russo C, Palaia G, Lo Giudice R, Vecchio AD, Visca P et al. Biopsy of Different Oral Soft Tissues Lesions by KTP and Diode Laser: *Histological Evaluation*. Hindawi *e Scientific World Journal* 2014.

[136] Giri D, Agarwal N, Sinha A, Srivastava S, Mishra A. Diode laser: In treatment of recurrent verrucous leukoplakia. *Contemporary Clinical Dentistry* Apr-Jun 2016; 7(2):250-254.

[137] Corso GD, Gissi DB, Tarsitano A, Costabile E, Marchetti C, Montebugnoli L et al. Laser evaporation versus laser excision of oral leukoplakia: A retrospective study with long-term follow-up. *Journal of Cranio-Maxillo-Facial Surgery* xxx (2015) 1e6.

[138] Chainani-Wu N, Lee D, Madden E, Sim C, Collins K, Silverman Jr S. Clinical predictors of oral leukoplakia recurrence following CO2 laser vaporization. *Journal of Cranio-Maxillo-Facial Surgery* 2015; 1-5.

[139] López-Jornet P, Camacho-Alonso F. Comparison of pain and swelling after removal of oral leukoplakia with CO_2 laser and cold knife: A randomized clinical trial. *Med Oral Patol Oral Cir Bucal.* 2013 Jan 1;18 (1):e38-44.

[140] Armenores P, James CL, Walker PC, Huilgol SC. Treatment of actinic cheilitis with the Er:YAG laser. *J am acad dermatol* October 2010; 63(4):642-646.

[141] de Godoy Peres FF, Brandão AAH, Carvalho YR, Filho UD, Plapler H. A study of actinic cheilitis treatment by two low morbidity CO_2 laser vaporization one-pass protocols. *Lasers Med* Sci 2009; 24:375–385.

[142] Cohen JL. Erbium laser resurfacing in actinic chelitis. *J Drugs Dermatol.* 2013 Nov; 12(11):1290-2.

[143] Castiñeiras I, DelPozo J, Mazaira M, Rodríguez-Lojo R. Actinic cheilitis: Evolution to squamous cell carcinoma after carbon dioxide laser vaporization. A study of 43 cases. *Journal of Dermatological Treatment*. 2010; 21:49–53.

[144] Calzavara-Pinton PG, Rossi MT, Sala R. A retrospective analysis of real-life practice of off-label photodynamic therapy using methyl aminolevulinate (MAL-PDT) in 20 Italian dermatology departments. Part 2: oncologic and infectious indications. *Photochem Photobiol Sci* 2013;12:158–65.

[145] Ribeiro CF, Souza FH, Jordão JM, Haendchen LC, et al. Photodynamic therapy in actinic cheilitis: clinical and anatomopathological evaluation of 19 patients. *An Bras Dermatol* 2012;87:418–23.

[146] Fai D, Romano I, Cassano N, Vena GA. Methyl-aminolevulinate photodynamic therapy for the treatment of actinic cheilitis: a retrospective evaluation of 29 patients. *G Ital Dermatol Venereol* 2012;147:99–101.

[147] Sotiriou E, Apalla Z, Chovarda E, Panagiotidou D, Ioannides D. Photodynamic therapy with 5-aminolevulinic acid in actinic cheilitis: an 18-month clinical and histological follow-up. *J Eur Acad Dermatol Venereol*. 2010 Aug;24(8):916-20.

[148] Castaño E, Comunión A, Arias D, Miñano R, Romero A, Borbujo J. Tratamiento de queilitis actínicas con terapia fotodinámica [Photodynamic therapy for actinic cheilitis]. *Actas Dermosifiliogr*. 2009 Dec;100(10):895-8. Spanish.

[149] Rossi R, Assad GB, Buggiani G, Lotti T. Photodynamic therapy: treatment of choice for actinic cheilitis? *Dermatol Ther* 2008;21:412–5.

[150] Zaiac M, Clement A. Treatment of actinic cheilitis by photodynamic therapy with 5-Aminolevulinic acid and blue light activation. *J Drugs Dermatol* 2011;10:1240–5.

[151] Sotiriou E, Apalla Z, Koussidou-Erremonti T, Ioannides D. Actinic cheilitis treated with one cycle of 5-aminolaevulinic acid-based photodynamic therapy: report of 10 cases. *Br J Dermatol* 2008;159: 261–2.

[152] Alexiades-Armenakas MR, Geronemus RG. Laser-mediated photodynamic therapy of actinic cheilitis. *J Drugs Dermatol* 2004;3:548–51.

[153] Choi SH, Kim KH, Song KH. Efficacy of ablative fractional laser-assisted photodynamic therapy for the treatment of actinic cheilitis: 12-month follow-up results of a prospective, randomized, comparative trial. *British Journal of Dermatology* (2015); 173:184–191.

[154] Yang SW, Leec YS, Chang LC, Hsieh TY, Chen TA. Outcome of excision of oral erythroplakia. *British Journal of Oral and Maxillofacial Surgery* 53 (2015) 142–147.

[155] Yamaguchi Y., et al. A case of erythroplasia of Queyrat successfully treated with combination carbon dioxide laser vaporization and surgery. *J Eur Acad Dermatol Venereol* 2014.

[156] Del Losada JP, Ferré A, San Román B, Vieira V, Fonseca E. Erythroplasia of Queyrat with urethral involvement: treatment with

carbon dioxide laser vaporization. *Dermatol Surg.* 2005 Nov;31(11 Pt 1):1454-7.

[157] Conejo-Mir JS, Muñoz MA, Linares M, Rodríguez L, Serrano A. Carbon dioxide laser treatment of erythroplasia of Queyrat: a revisited treatment to this condition. *J Eur Acad Dermatol Venereol.* 2005 Sep;19(5):643-4.

[158] Van Bezooijen BP, Horenblas S, Meinhardt W, Newling DW. Laser therapy for carcinoma in situ of the penis. *J Urol.* 2001 Nov;166(5):1670-1.

[159] Nouri K. *Lasers in Dermatology and Medicine*; 2012. doi:10.1007/978-0-85729-281-0.

[160] Calzavara-Pinton PG, Rossi MT, Aronson E, Sala R; Italian Group For Photodynamic Therapy. A retrospective analysis of real-life practice of off-label photodynamic therapy using methyl aminolevulinate (MAL-PDT) in 20 Italian dermatology departments. Part 1: inflammatory and aesthetic indications. *Photochem Photobiol Sci.* 2013 Jan;12(1):148-57.

[161] Park JY, Kim SJ, Kim YC. Erythroplasia of Queyrat refractory to photodynamic therapy. *Clin Exp Dermatol* 2012; 37(7):795-797.

[162] Fai D, Romano I, Cassano N, Vena GA. Methyl-aminolevulinate photodynamic therapy for the treatment of erythroplasia of Queyrat in 23 patients. *J Dermatolog Treat.* 2012 Oct;23(5):330-2.

[163] Paoli J, Ternesten Bratel A, Löwhagen GB, Stenquist B, Forslund O, Wennberg AM. Penile intraepithelial neoplasia: results of photodynamic therapy. *Acta Derm Venereol.* 2006;86(5):418-21.

[164] Wang XL, Wang HW, Guo MX, Xu SZ. Treatment of skin cancer and pre-cancer using topical ALA-PDT--a single hospital experience. *Photodiagnosis Photodyn Ther.* 2008 Jun;5(2):127-33.

[165] Strauss RA: Laser management of discrete lesions. In Catone G, Alling C, editors: *Laser applications in oral and maxillofacial surgery,* Philadelphia, 1997, Saunders.

[166] Draganova-Filipova MN, Zagorchev PI and Tomov GT. Effects of Low Level Laser Therapy on Erosive-atrophic *Oral Lichen Planus.* Folia Medica 2018; 60(3): 417-423.

[167] Liu WB, Sun LW, Yang H, Wang YF. Treatment of oral lichen planus using 308-nm excimer laser. *Dermatologic Therapy*. 2017; e12510: 1-3.

[168] Akram Z, Abduljabbar T, Vohra F, Javed F. *Efficacy of low level laser therapy compared to steroid therapy in the treatment of oral lichen planus: A systematic review.*

[169] Mücke T, Gentz I, Kanatas A, Ritschl LM, Mitchell DA, Wolff KD et al. Clinical trial analyzing the impact of continuous defocused CO_2 laser vaporisation on the malignant transformation of erosive oral lichen planus. *Journal of Cranio-Maxillo-Facial Surgery* 2015; xxx 1e4: 1-4.

[170] Cafaro A, Arduino PG, Massolini GL, Romagnoli E, Broccoletti R. Clinical evaluation of the efficiency of low-level laser therapy for oral lichen planus: a prospective case series. *Lasers Med Sci* 2014; 29:185–190.

[171] Agha-Hosseini F, Moslemi E, Mirzaii-Dizgah I. Comparative evaluation of low level laser and CO_2 laser in treatment of patients with oral lichen planus. *Int. J. Oral Maxillofac. Surg*. 2012; 41: 1265–1269.

[172] Pavlić V, Vujic-Aleksic V. Phototherapy approaches in treatment of oral lichen planus. *Photodermatology Photoimmunology and Photomedicine* 2013; 30(1): 15-24.

[173] Choi SH, Kim KH, Song KH. Efficacy of ablative fractional laser-assisted photodynamic therapy for the treatment of actinic cheilitis: 12-month follow-up results of a prospective, randomised, comparative trial. *British Journal of Dermatology* 2015; 173(1): 184-191.

[174] Bargiela-Pérez P, González-Merchán J, Díaz-Sánchez R, Serrera-Figallo MA,Volland G, Joergens M, et al. Prospective study of the 532 nm laser (KTP) versus diode laser 980 nm in the resection of hyperplastic lesions of the oral cavity. *Med Oral Patol Oral Cir Bucal.* 2018 Jan 1; 23 (1):e78 85.

[175] Yamaguchi T, Shindoh M, Amemiya A, Inoue N, Kawamura M, Sakaoka H, et al. Detection of human papillomavirus type 2 related sequence in oral papilloma. *Anal Cell Pathol.* 1998; 16(3):125–30.

[176] Eversole L. Papillary lesions of the oral cavity: relationship to human papillomaviruses. *J Calif Dent Assoc.* 2000; 28(12):922–927.

[177] Rakhewar PS, Patil HP, Thorat MK. Diode laser treatment of an oral squamous papilloma of soft palate. *Journal of Dental Lasers.* 2015; 2(9): 114-117.

[178] Leffell DJ, Braverman IM. Familial multiple lipomatosis: report of a case and a review of the literature. *J Am Acad Dermatol.* 1986; 15(2):275–279.

[179] Jafarzadeh H, Sanatkhani M, Mohtasham N. Oral pyogenic granuloma: a review. *J Oral Sci.* 2006;48(4):167–175.

[180] Wyrębek B, Orzechowska A, Cudziło D, Plakwicz P. Evaluation of changes in the width of gingiva in children and youth. Review of literature. *Dev Period Med.* 2015 Apr-Jun;19(2):212-6.

[181] Romanos G, Nentwig G-H. Diode laser (980 nm) in oral and maxillofacial surgical procedures: clinical observations based on clinical applications. *J Clin Laser Med Surg.* 1999;17(5):193–7.

[182] de Serres LM, Sie KC, Richardson MA. Lymphatic malformations of the head and neck. A proposal for staging. *Arch Otolaryngol Head Neck Surg.* 1995;121:577–82.

[183] Bozkaya S, Dilek Ug, Ceylan SU, et al. The treatment of lymphangioma in the buccal mucosa by radiofrequency ablation: a case report. *Oral Surg Oral Med Oral Pathol Oral Radiol Endod* 2006; 102: e28–e31.

[184] Claesson G, Kuylenstierna R. OK-432 therapy for lymphatic malformation in 32 patients. *Pediatr Otorhinolaryngol Int J* 2002; 65: 1–6.

[185] Mechery R, Kumar M, Arora P, Dinakar N. Lymphangioma of lip treated with carbon dioxide laser. *Journal of Dental Lasers.* 2016; 2(10) : 81-84.

[186] Frame JW. Carbon dioxide laser surgery for benign oral lesions. *Br Dent J* 1985; 158(4): 125–128.

[187] Jinbu Y, Kusama M, Itoh H, Matsumoto K, Wang J, Noguchi T. Mucocele of the glands of Blandin-Nuhn: clinical and histopathologic analysis of 26 cases. *Oral Surg Oral Med Oral Pathol Oral Radiol Endod* 2003; 95(4): 467–470.

[188] Kopp WK, St-Hilaire H. Mucosal preservation in the treatment of mucocele with CO_2 laser. *J Oral Maxillofac Surg* 2004; 62(12): 1559–1561.

[189] Niccoli-Filho W, Morosolli AR. Surgical treatment of ranula with carbon dioxide laser radiation. *Lasers Med Sci* 2004; 19(1): 12–14.

[190] Bornstein MM, Winzap-Kälin C, Cochran DL, Buser D. The CO2 laser for excisional biopsies of oral lesions: a case series study. Int *J Periodontics Restorative Dent* 2005; 25(3): 221–229.

[191] Zola M, Rosenberg D, Anakwa K. Treatment of a ranula using an Er,Cr:YSGG laser. *J Oral Maxillofac Surg*. 2006; 64(5): 823–827.

[192] Kato J, Wijeyeweera RL. The effect of CO(2) laser irradiation on oral soft tissue problems in children in Sri Lanka. *Photomed Laser Surg* 2007; 25(4): 264–268.

[193] Huang IY, Chen CM, Kao YH, Worthington P. Treatment of mucocele of the lower lip with carbon dioxide laser. *J Oral Maxillofac Surg* 2007; 65(5): 855–858.

[194] Yagüe-García J, España-Tost AJ, Berini-Aytés L, Gay-Escoda C. Treatment of oral mucocele-scalpel versus CO_2 laser. *Med Oral Pathol Oral Cir Buccal* 2009; 14(9): e469–474.

[195] Boj JR, Poirier C, Espasa E, Hernandez M, Espanya A. Lower lip mucocele treated with an erbium laser. *Pediatr Dent* 2009; 31(3): 249–252.

[196] Pedron IG, Galletta VC, Azevedo LH, Corrêa L. Treatment of mucocele of the lower lip with diode laser in pediatric patients: presentation of 2 clinical cases. *Pediatr Dent* 2010; 32(7): 539–541.

[197] Huang IY, Chen CM, Kao YH, Worthington P. Treatment of mucocele of the lower lip with carbon dioxide laser. *J Oral Maxillofac Surg* 2007; 65(5): 855–858.

[198] Frame JW. Carbon dioxide laser surgery for benign oral lesions. *Br Dent J* 1985; 158(4): 125–128.

[199] Jinbu Y, Kusama M, Itoh H, Matsumoto K, Wang J, Noguchi T. Mucocele of the glands of Blandin-Nuhn: clinical and histopathologic analysis of 26 cases. *Oral Surg Oral Med Oral Pathol Oral Radiol Endod* 2003; 95(4): 467–470.

[200] Kopp WK, St-Hilaire H. Mucosal preservation in the treatment of mucocele with CO_2 laser. *J Oral Maxillofac Surg* 2004; 62(12):1559–1561.

[201] Niccoli-Filho W, Morosolli AR. Surgical treatment of ranula with carbon dioxide laser radiation. *Lasers Med Sci* 2004; 19(1): 12–14.

[202] Bornstein MM, Winzap-Kälin C, Cochran DL, Buser D. The CO_2 laser for excisional biopsies of oral lesions: a case series study. *Int J Periodontics Restorative Dent* 2005; 25(3): 221–229.

[203] Zola M, Rosenberg D, Anakwa K. Treatment of a ranula using an Er,Cr:YSGG laser. *J Oral Maxillofac Surg*. 2006; 64(5): 823–827.

[204] Kato J, Wijeyeweera RL. The effect of CO(2) laser irradiation on oral soft tissue problems in children in Sri Lanka. *Photomed Laser Surg* 2007; 25(4): 264–268.

[205] Huang IY, Chen CM, Kao YH, Worthington P. Treatment of mucocele of the lower lip with carbon dioxide laser. *J Oral Maxillofac Surg* 2007; 65(5): 855–858.

[206] Yagüe-García J, España-Tost AJ, Berini-Aytés L, Gay-Escoda C. Treatment of oral mucocele-scalpel versus CO_2 laser. *Med Oral Pathol Oral Cir Buccal* 2009; 14(9): e469–474.

[207] Boj JR, Poirier C, Espasa E, Hernandez M, Espanya A. Lower lip mucocele treated with an erbium laser. *Pediatr Dent* 2009; 31(3): 249–252.

[208] Pedron IG, Galletta VC, Azevedo LH, Corrêa L. Treatment of mucocele of the lower lip with diode laser in pediatric patients:

presentation of 2 clinical cases. *Pediatr Dent* 2010; 32(7): 539–541.

[209] Mohanraj M, Prabhu VR, Senthil R. Diagnostic Methods for Early Detection of Dental Caries – A Review. *International Journal of Pedodontic Rehabilitation* 2016; 1(1): 29-36.

[210] Gazelius B, Olgart L, Edwall B, Edwall L. Non-invasive recording of blood flow in human dental pulp. *Endod Dent Traumatol.* 1986;2:219–21.

[211] Olgart L, Gazelius B, Lindh-Strömberg U. Laser Doppler flowmetry in assessing vitality in luxated permanent teeth. *Int Endod J.* 1988;21:300–6.

[212] Andreasen FM, Andreasen JO. Luxation injuries. In: Andreasen JO, Andreasen FM, editors. *Textbook and color Atlas of traumatic injuries to the teeth.* 3rd ed. Copenhagen: Munksgaard; 1994. p. 353–4.

[213] Ebihara A, Tokita Y, Izawa T, Suda H. Pulpal blood flow assessed by laser Doppler flowmetry in a tooth with a horizontal root fracture. *Oral Surg Oral Med Oral Pathol Oral Radiol Endod.* 1996;81:229–33.

[214] Ikawa M, Komatsu H, Ikawa K, Mayanagi H, Shimauchi H. Age-related changes in the human pulpal blood flow measured by laser Doppler flowmetry. *Dent Traumatol.* 2003;19:36–40.

[215] Babacan H, Doruk C, Bicakci AA. Pulpal blood flow changes due to rapid maxillary expansion. *Angle Orthod.* 2010;80:1136–40.

[216] Cho JJ, Efstratiadis S, Hasselgren G. Pulp vitality after rapid palatal expansion. *Am J Orthod Dentofacial Orthop.* 2010; 137:254–8.

[217] Reddy, Praveen. Optical coherence tomography in the diagnosis of oral cancer. *Journal of Cancer Research and Therapeutics* 2017; 13(6):883-888.

[218] Shivhare P, Shankarnarayan L, Basavaraju SM, Yadav M, Singh A. Optical Coherence Tomography; A Modern Technique to Detect Oral Mucosal Lesion: A Review. *IJSS Case Reports & Reviews* 2015; 1(12):51-54.

[219] Popescu DP, Choo-Smith LP, Flueraru C, Mao Y, Chang S, Disano J et al. Optical coherence tomography: fundamental principles, instrumental designs and biomedical applications. *Biophys Rev* (2011) 3:155–169.

[220] Liu D, Zhao X, Zeng X, Dan H, Chen Q. Non-Invasive Techniques for Detection and Diagnosis of Oral Potentially Malignant Disorders. Tohoku *J. Exp. Med.* 2016; 238:165-177.

[221] Sahu, Krishna. Optical diagnostics in oral cancer: An update on Raman spectroscopic Applications. *Journal of Cancer Research and Therapeutics* 2017; 13(6):908-915.

[222] Chandra S, Sah K. Spectroscopy: A New Diagnostic Technique for Detection of Potentially Malignant Oral Lesions. *Journal of Indian Academy of Oral Medicine and Radiology* 2010;22(3):144-146.

[223] Stone N, Stavroulaki P, Kendall C, Birchall M, Barr H. Raman spectroscopy for early detection of laryngeal malignancy: Preliminary results. *Laryngoscope* 2000;110:1756-63.

[224] Lau DP, Huang Z, Lui H, Man CS, Berean K, et al. Raman spectroscopy for optical diagnosis in normal and cancerous tissue of the nasopharynx preliminary findings. *Lasers Surg Med* 2003;32:210-14.

[225] Malini R, Venkatakrishna K, Kurien J, Pai KM, Rao L, et al. Discrimination of normal, inflammatory, premalignant, and malignant oral tissue: A raman spectroscopy study. *Biopolymers* 2006;81:179-93.

[226] Fulwyler MJ. Electronic separation of biological cells by volume. *Science* 1965; 150: 910–911.

[227] Perfetto SP, Chattopadhyay PK, Roederer M. Seventeen-colour flow cytometry: unravelling the immune system. *Nat. Rev. Immunol.* 2004; 4:648–655.

[228] Macey, M. G. (Ed.). *Flow cytometry: Principles and applications*. Totowa, NJ: Humana Press 2007.

[229] Ibrahim SF, van den Engh, G. Flow cytometry and cell sorting. *Advances in Biochemical Engineering/Biotechnology* 2007; 106:19–39.

[230] Mach WJ, Thimmesch AR, Orr JA, Slusser J G, Pierce JD. Flow cytometry and laser scanning cytometry, a comparison of techniques. *Journal of Clinical Monitoring and Computing* 2010; 24: 251–259.

[231] Betters DM. Use of Flow Cytometry in Clinical Practice. *J Adv Pract Oncol* 2015;6:435–440.

[232] Han Y, Gu Y, Zhang AC, Lo YH. Review: imaging technologies for flow cytometry. *The Royal Society of Chemistry* 2016;16:4639–4647.

[233] Raju T B V G, Garapati S, Agrawal R, Reddy S, Razdan A, Kumar SK. Sterilizing Endodontic Files by four different sterilization methods to prevent cross-infection - An *In-vitro* Study. *Journal of International Oral Health*. Nov-Dec 2013; 5(6):108-12.

About the Authors

Fakir Mohan Debta graduated from SCB Dental College, Cuttack in the year 2000. He obtained his post graduation degree in the branch of Oral Medicine and Radiology, from Government Dental College and Hospital, Ahmedabad, Gujarat University, in the year 2004. With almost 17 years of teaching experience, he is currently working in the capacity of Professor and Head of the Department of Oral Medicine and Radiology, Cuttack, Odisha, India. An eminent academician and skilful oral diagnostician, he specializes in early diagnosis and prompt conservative therapy of oral and maxillofacial lesions. He is one of the first in his state to explore the role of lasers as a diagnostic and adjunctive therapeutic tool in the field of oral and maxillofacial medicine. His astute thinking and clinical judgments make him one of the most reckoned for oral and maxillofacial diagnostician and radiologist of his time.

Ekagrata Mishra graduated from SCB Dental College, Cuttack in the year 2016 and completed her post-graduation from the same institute in the branch of Oral Medicine and Radiology in the year 2020. She is currently working as a Post-PG Resident in the Department of Oral Medicine and Radiology, SCB Dental College and Hospital, Cuttack, Odisha.

Neha Patyal graduated from Dr. Harvansh Singh Judge Institute of Dental Sciences and Hospital, Chandigarh, in the year 2013 and completed her-post graduation from SCB Dental College and Hospital in the discipline of Public Health Dentistry in the year 2020. She is currently working as a Post-PG Resident in the Department of Public Health Dentistry, SCB Dental College and Hospital, Cuttack, Odisha.

INDEX

G

H

I

J

K

L

M

N

O

P

Q

R

S

T

U

V

W

Y

α

β